T0206071

SpringerBriefs in Statistics

JSS Research Series in Statistics

The current research of statistics in Japan has expanded in several directions in line with recent trends in academic activities in the area of statistics and statistical sciences over the globe. The core of these research activities in statistics in Japan has been the Japan Statistical Society (JSS). This society, the oldest and largest academic organization for statistics in Japan, was founded in 1931 by a handful of pioneer statisticians and economists and now has a history of about 80 years. Many distinguished scholars have been members, including the influential statistician Hirotugu Akaike, who was a past president of JSS, and the notable mathematician Kiyosi Itô, who was an earlier member of the Institute of Statistical Mathematics (ISM), which has been a closely related organization since the establishment of ISM. The society has two academic journals: the Journal of the Japan Statistical Society (English Series) and the Journal of the Japan Statistical Society (Japanese Series). The membership of JSS consists of researchers, teachers, and professional statisticians in many different fields including mathematics, statistics, engineering, medical sciences, government statistics, economics, business, psychology, education, and many other natural, biological, and social sciences.

The JSS Series of Statistics aims to publish recent results of current research activities in the areas of statistics and statistical sciences in Japan that otherwise would not be available in English; they are complementary to the two JSS academic journals, both English and Japanese. Because the scope of a research paper in academic journals inevitably has become narrowly focused and condensed in recent years, this series is intended to fill the gap between academic research activities and the form of a single academic paper.

The series will be of great interest to a wide audience of researchers, teachers, professional statisticians, and graduate students in many countries who are interested in statistics and statistical sciences, in statistical theory, and in various areas of statistical applications.

More information about this series at http://www.springer.com/series/13497

Akihiro Hirakawa · Hiroyuki Sato
Takashi Daimon · Shigeyuki Matsui

Modern Dose-Finding Designs for Cancer Phase I Trials: Drug Combinations and Molecularly Targeted Agents

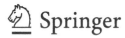 Springer

Akihiro Hirakawa
Department of Biostatistics
and Bioinformatics, Graduate
School of Medicine
The University of Tokyo
Tokyo
Japan

Hiroyuki Sato
Pharmaceuticals and Medical
Devices Agency
Tokyo
Japan

Takashi Daimon
Division of Biostatistics
Hyogo College of Medicine
Nishinomiya, Hyogo
Japan

Shigeyuki Matsui
Department of Biostatistics, Graduate
School of Medicine
Nagoya University
Nagoya, Aichi
Japan

ISSN 2191-544X   ISSN 2191-5458   (electronic)
SpringerBriefs in Statistics
ISSN 2364-0057   ISSN 2364-0065   (electronic)
JSS Research Series in Statistics
ISBN 978-4-431-55572-8   ISBN 978-4-431-55573-5   (eBook)
https://doi.org/10.1007/978-4-431-55573-5

Library of Congress Control Number: 2018930526

Printed on acid-free paper

This Springer imprint is published by the registered company Springer Japan KK part of Springer Nature
The registered company address is: Shiroyama Trust Tower, 4-3-1 Toranomon, Minato-ku, Tokyo
105-6005, Japan

To our beloved families and ex-colleagues/colleagues at the University of Tokyo, Pharmaceuticals and Medical Devices Agency, Hyogo College of Medicine, and Nagoya University.

Preface

Novel treatments of cancers have emerged over the past decade. Along with this growing trend, innovative phase I trial designs for determining a maximum tolerated dose (MTD) or recommended phase 2 dose (RP2D) have also been devised. In contrast to the emergence of such statistical dose-finding approaches, most phase I trials have a classic dose escalation design such as the 3 + 3 scheme in practice because of its ease of use. Because the utility of the innovative dose-finding designs has been examined in a large number of studies, we need to get away from the comfort zone of application of the classic dose escalation designs to increase the success rate of anticancer drug development. The aim of this book is to contribute to the modernization of dose-finding methods in phase I trials by describing statistical methodologies of recent innovative dose-finding methods as well as their user-friendly software implementations.

This book deals with advanced methods for phase I dose-finding clinical trials with multiple drugs and/or outcomes in oncology. In addition to the methodological aspects of the dose-finding methods, the text also provides software implementations and practical considerations for applying these complex methods to real cancer clinical trials. Thus, in this book, we aim to provide researchers working in biostatistics and other statistical sciences a good summary of recent developments in complex dose-finding methods as well as to offer practitioners in biostatistics and clinical investigators advanced information for designing, conducting, monitoring, and analyzing complex dose-finding trials. The topics in the book are mainly related to cancer clinical trials, but many are potentially applicable or extendable to trials dealing with other diseases.

The book mainly focuses on model-based dose-finding methods for two kinds of phase I trials. One is clinical trials of a combination of two agents. When developing dose-finding methods for two-agent combination trials, we need reasonable models that can adequately capture joint toxicity probabilities for two agents, taking into consideration possible interactions of the two agents on toxicity probability (e.g., synergistic or antagonistic effects). The other is clinical trials evaluating both efficacy and toxicity outcomes in single- and two-agent combination trials. These methods are often applied to the phase I trials of molecularly targeted agents

(MTAs) because the toxicity and efficacy for an MTA do not monotonically increase with the dose, but the efficacy often increases initially with the dose and then plateaus. Successful software implementations for several dose-finding methods we introduced in this book are shown and their practical operating characteristics are discussed. Recent topics on dose-finding methods for MTAs are also elaborated.

Chapter 1 provides key points of phase I cancer trials. We also overview the 3 + 3 design as a rule-based dose-finding method and then a continual reassessment method (CRM) as a model-based dose-finding method for monotherapy (i.e., the use of a single agent). Chapter 2 is devoted to the dose-finding methods for two-agent combination trials. In two-agent combination phase I trials, we need to capture the dose–toxicity relationship for combination of two agents and to identify MTD combinations of the two agents. We compared several rival methods and summarized the operating characteristics of each method. Chapter 3 introduces dose-finding designs that determine the optimal dose based on the joint assessment of toxicity and efficacy of an agent. Various types of incorporation of toxicity and efficacy outcomes into dose-finding methods have been developed. We discuss four Bayesian designs in this chapter. Chapter 4 describes dose-finding methods for MTAs to determine the optimal dose in singe-agent trials. Finally, we introduce some recent advanced topics on dose-finding designs including seamless phase I/II trials, designs that account for late-onset toxicity and efficacy outcomes, dose finding based on relative dose intensity, cancer immunotherapy, and dose individualization for precision medicine in Chap. 5.

Finally, we are grateful for a Grant-in-Aid for Scientific Research (Nos. 16H06299, 15K15948, 15K00058, and 17K00045) from the Ministry of Education, Culture, Sports, Science and Technology of Japan for supporting this book project. The views expressed here are the result of an independent study and do not represent the viewpoints or findings of the Pharmaceuticals and Medical Devices Agency.

Tokyo, Japan   Akihiro Hirakawa
November 2017   Hiroyuki Sato
                                                                                    Takashi Daimon
                                                                                    Shigeyuki Matsui

Contents

Acronyms

BMA   Bayesian model averaging
CRM   Continual reassessment method
MTA   Molecularly targeted agent
MTD   Maximum tolerated dose
RP2D   Recommended phase 2 dose

Chapter 1
Dose Finding in Phase I Cancer Trials

Abstract The objective of phase I cancer trials is to determine the optimal dose of an agent or a combination of agents that can serve as a recommended phase 2 dose (RP2D). The conventionally defined RP2D of a cytotoxic agent corresponds to the maximum tolerated dose (MTD), defined as the highest dose with acceptable toxicity. MTD is generally calculated from dose-limiting toxicity data obtained during the first, and rarely, the second cycle of treatment. The dose-finding methods for determining the MTD are roughly categorized into two groups: (1) those based on prespecified dose escalation or de-escalation rules; and (2) those based on a statistical dose–response model. In contrast to cytotoxic agents, the RP2D of molecularly targeted agents (MTAs) may not be necessarily identical to their MTD owing to the mechanism of action. Therefore, the reasonable dose-finding methods for determining the RP2D of cytotoxic agents and of MTAs are considered different. This introductory chapter provides key points on phase I cancer trials and an overview the rule-and model-based dose-finding methods for monotherapy (i.e., the use of a single agent) that are the prototype of all the innovative dose-finding methods developed recently.

Keywords Dose finding · Maximum tolerated dose · Phase I · Recommended phase 2 dose

1.1 Cytotoxic Agents and MTAs

Cytotoxic agents are those aimed at directly killing cancer cells. Nonetheless, they also kill other cells likewise, such as normal cells, as a systemic action, and therefore they may have serious adverse effects. Thus, it is thought that the efficacy and toxicity of cytotoxic agents stem from the same biological mechanism, closely linked to each other. In addition, for cytotoxic agents, it is natural to consider an assumption of monotonicity, where higher doses may yield greater efficacy but lesser safety. In general, the fatal nature of the disease may allow for the use of an MTD, in hopes of killing all cancer cells. This approach is behind the strategy of traditional early-phase clinical trials for cytotoxic agents. The aim is to determine the MTD based

© The Author(s), under exclusive licence to Springer Japan KK, part of Springer Nature 2018   1
A. Hirakawa et al., *Modern Dose-Finding Designs for Cancer Phase I Trials: Drug Combinations and Molecularly Targeted Agents*, JSS Research Series in Statistics, https://doi.org/10.1007/978-4-431-55573-5_1

on toxicity data in a phase I trial, followed by evaluation of efficacy at MTD in a subsequent phase II trial.

MTAs differ from standard chemotherapy in several ways. MTAs block the growth and spread of a tumor by interfering with specific molecules ("molecular targets") that are involved in the growth, progression, and spread of the tumor, whereas most of cytotoxic agents act on all rapidly dividing normal and cancerous cells. MTAs are also deliberately chosen or designed to interact with their target, whereas many cytotoxic agents have been identified because they kill cells. MTAs are often cytostatic (that is, they block tumor cell proliferation); therefore, the dose–efficacy curves of MTAs do not always monotonically increase with the dose escalation. Jain et al. (2010) concluded that targeted agents may have different dose–response relationships as compared with cytotoxic chemotherapies. Le Tourneau et al. (2010) suggested that some MTAs do not necessarily need to be administered at their MTD to obtain maximal efficacy. In the determination of an optimal dose for MTAs, dose-finding methods that take into account the bivariate-correlating outcomes of both efficacy and toxicity are required.

1.2 Classification of Phase I Cancer Trials

The objective of phase I cancer trials is to determine the optimal dose of an agent or a combination of agents that can serve as the RP2D. The secondary objectives are to evaluate the toxicity including dose-limiting toxicity, pharmacokinetics, and the antitumor effect in the schedule under evaluation. The conventionally defined RP2D of a cytotoxic agent corresponds to the MTD, defined as the highest dose with acceptable toxicity. MTD is generally determined from dose-limiting toxicity data obtained during the first, and rarely, the second cycle of treatment. In two-agent combination phase I trials, investigators need to capture the dose–toxicity relationship for combination of two agents and identify MTD combinations of the two agents. The dose-finding methods for determining the MTD (or MTD combination) are roughly categorized into two groups: (1) those based on prespecified dose escalation or de-escalation rules; and (2) those based on a statistical dose–response model.

In contrast to cytotoxic agents, the RP2D of MTAs may not necessarily be identical to their MTD owing to the mechanism of action. Therefore, dose-finding methods that take account the efficacy outcome in addition to the toxicity outcome are warranted for the clinical development of MTAs. The dose–efficacy model for MTAs is necessary to capture the specific relation between efficacy and a dose level. The efficacy may increase initially with the dose level but then reaches a plateau; however, this may not always be the case. Several powerful methods were developed recently. Thus, the reasonable dose-finding methods for determining the RP2D of cytotoxic agents and MTAs are considered to be different.

Before introducing the statistical methodologies for recent innovative dose-finding methods for a combination therapy of two agents and MTAs, we first overview the rule- and model-based dose-finding methods for monotherapy (i.e., the use of a single agent) that are the prototype of all the innovative dose-finding methods developed recently. Eisenhauer et al. (2015) described the basics of dose-finding designs including the 3 + 3 designs as well as information on the process, pitfalls, and logistics of phase I trials. Cheung (2011) focused on the theory and application of the continual reassessment method (CRM). Statistical properties and operating characteristics of rule- and model-based dose-finding methods have been examined in several studies (e.g., O'Quigley and Chevret 1991, Chevret 1993, Lin and Shih 2001, Iasonos et al. 2008).

1.3   Rule-Based Methods

1.3.1   3 + 3 Design

The most well-known and widely used rule-based method is the 3 + 3 design (Carter 1973; Storer 1989). This design enrolls a group of three patients and treats them with the starting (usually, the lowest) dose level. Based on the observed prespecified toxicity (usually, dose-limiting toxicity), we determine the dose level allocated to the next cohort of patients and the MTD as follows:

Step 1:   Treat three patients at the starting dose level and observe the toxicities.

(a) If none of the three patients develops toxicity, then allocate the next higher dose to the next cohort of patients, and repeat Step 1.
(b) If one out of three patients experiences toxicity, then go to Step 2.
(c) If at least two out of three patients experience toxicity, then go to Step 3.

Step 2:   Treat three more patients at the same dose level and observe the toxicities.

(a) If one out of the six patients experiences toxicity, then allocate the next higher dose to the next cohort of patients and go to Step 1.
(b) If at least two out of the six patients experience toxicity, then go to Step 3.

Step 3:   Stop dose escalation, and the next lower dose level is generally selected as the MTD.

Figure 1.1 shows an example of dose assignment for the 3 + 3 design.

1.3.2   Other Relevant Methods

Accelerated-titration designs proposed by Simon et al. (1997) are also a widely used rule-based method. The main features of this design are (i) to include a rapid

Fig. 1.1 Dose assignment for the 3 + 3 design

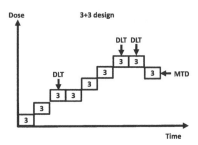

initial escalation stage, called an accelerated stage, where one patient per dose level is treated, (ii) to account for moderate toxicity in addition to the dose-limiting toxicity, (iii) to have options to use intrapatient dose modification, and (iv) to analyze trial results by means of the model that incorporates parameters for intra- and interpatient variation in toxicity and cumulative toxicity. They compared the operating characteristics of the 3 + 3 design with those of the three different designs with an accelerated phase. In addition, the best-of-5 design (Storer 2001) and the rolling six design (Skolnik et al. 2008) may be useful in practice.

1.4 Model-Based Methods

1.4.1 Bayesian CRM

The most well-known model-based method is the CRM developed by the O'Quigley et al. (1990). The CRM is the well-established prototype of the various recent model-based methods. The CRM involves a dose–toxicity model and estimates the model parameters based on the Bayesian theorem. For patient i, if a predefined toxicity is observed, primarily the dose-limiting toxicity, we denote $Y_i = 1$; otherwise, $Y_i = 0$. We let $\Pr\{Y_i = 1\}$ be the probability that $Y_i = 1$, often modeling this probability using a one-parameter logistic regression model with a fixed intercept β_0:

$$\Pr\{Y_i = 1\} = \psi(x_i \mid \beta_1) = \frac{\exp(\beta_0 + \beta_1 x_i)}{1 + \exp(\beta_0 + \beta_1 x_i)}, \tag{1.1}$$

where x_i is the dose level of an agent for patient i, and β_1 is the regression coefficient. O'Quigley et al. (1990) also introduced alternate models, including power and hyperbolic tangent models. It should be noted that the numerical dose label x_is in the CRM is not necessarily the actual dose administered, but rather is defined on a conceptual scale that represents an ordering of the risks of toxicity based on initial guesses about toxicity probabilities, for example, *skeleton*.

In the original CRM, the first patient is allocated to the dose level initially believed to have toxicity closest to the target toxicity probability ϕ. After obtaining the data on the toxicity outcomes from the first j patients, $D_j = \{y_1, \cdots, y_j\}$, the CRM updates the posterior estimates of toxicity probabilities for the dose levels through the estimation of the posterior probability distribution $p_{j+1}(\beta_1|D_j)$ to determine the dose level allocated to the $(j+1)$th patient as follows:

$$p_{j+1}(\beta_1|D_j) = \frac{L_j(\beta_1|D_j)p(\beta_1)}{\int_{-\infty}^{\infty} L_j(\beta_1|D_j)p(\beta_1)d\beta_1}, \tag{1.2}$$

where $L_j(\beta_1|D_j)$ is the likelihood function of Eq. (1.1) for j patients; that is,

$$L_j(\beta_1|D_j) = \prod_{i=1}^{j}\{\psi(x_i \mid \beta_1)^{y_i}\}\{1 - \psi(x_i \mid \beta_1)^{(1-y_i)}\}, \tag{1.3}$$

and $p(\beta_1)$ is the prior probability distribution for β_1. In this simple one-parameter setting, the posterior estimate of β_1 may be most easily computed by a standard numerical quadrature method (e.g., trapezoidal rule), but computer-intensive simulation-based methods, such as the Markov chain Monte Carlo method, have been widely applied. Using the posterior mean of β_1, the posterior estimates of toxicity probabilities for the dose levels were obtained. The dose level (at which posterior toxicity probability is the closest to the target value ϕ) was then determined, and the $(j+1)$th patient was allocated to that dose level. Thus, dose allocation based on the posterior toxicity probability was performed until the maximum sample size $N_{\max}$ was reached. Eventually, the dose level with a posterior toxicity probability closest to the target value ϕ at the end of the trial was selected as MTD. Figure 1.2 shows the trace plot of dose assignment for the Bayesian CRM.

Practical performance of the CRM can be improved by introducing a safety stopping rule, by limiting each dose escalation to one level, and by treating patients in cohorts (Goodman et al. 1995). When treating in cohorts of three using the same dose level within the cohort, the first three patients are allocated to the lowest dose level in practice owing to ethical considerations. Cheung (2011) provided comprehensive reviews and extensive discussions of the CRM.

Fig. 1.2 Dose assignment for the Bayesian CRM

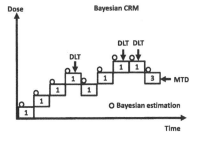

1.4.2   Other Relevant Designs

Babb et al. (1998) developed a dose-finding method that includes the escalation with overdose control on the basis of the Bayesian CRM. In this design, the expected proportion of patients treated at doses higher than the MTD is equal to a fixed level, α. Ji et al. (2007) proposed a simple dose-finding method that uses a beta/binomial model and a dose assignment rule based on posterior toxicity probabilities. Ji et al. (2010) devised the modified toxicity probability interval method by introducing the unit of probability mass that, given an interval and a probability distribution, is defined as the ratio of the probability mass of the interval to the length of the interval. Liu and Yuan (2015) additionally proposed an optimal Bayesian interval design that determines the dose escalation or de-escalation for the next cohorts of patients on the basis of the observed toxicity rate while minimizing the decision error of dose assignment.

References

Babb, J., Rogatko, A., Zacks, S.: Cancer phase I clinical trials: efficient dose escalation with overdose control. Stat. Med. **17**, 1103–1120 (1998)

Carter, S.K.: Study design principles for the clinical evaluation of new drugs as developed by the chemotherapy program of the National Cancer Institute. In: Staquet, M.J. (ed.) The Design of Clinical Trials in Cancer Therapy, pp. 242–289. Editions Scientifiques Europrennes, Brussels (1973)

Cheung, Y.K.: Dose Finding by the Continual Reassessment Method. Chapman and Hall, London (2011)

Chevret, S.: The continual reassessment method in cancer phase I clinical trials: A simulation study. Stat. Med. **12**, 1093–1108 (1993)

Eisenhauer, E.A., Twelves, C., Buyse, M.: Phase I Cancer Clinical Trials: A Practical Guide. Oxford University Press, New York (2015)

Goodman, S.N., Zahurak, M.L., Piantadosi, S.: Some practical improvements in the continual reassessment method for phase I studies. Stat. Med. **14**, 1149–1161 (1995)

Iasonos, A., Wilton, A.S., Riedel, E.R., Seshan, V.E., Spriggs, D.R.: A comprehensive comparison of the continual reassessment method to the standard 3 + 3 dose escalation scheme in phase I dose-finding studies. Clin. Trials **5**, 465–477 (2008)

Jain, R.K., Lee, J.J., Hong, D., Markman, M., Gong, J., Naing, A., Wheler, J., Kurzrock, R.: Phase I oncology studies: evidence that in the era of targeted therapies patients on lower doses do not fare worse. Clin. Cancer Res. **16**, 1289–97 (2010)

Ji, Y., Li, Y., Bekele, B.N.: Dose-finding in oncology clinical trials based on toxicity probability intervals. Clin. Trials **4**, 235–244 (2007)

Ji, Y., Liu, P., Li, Y., Bekele, B.N.: A modified toxicity probability interval method for dose-finding trials. Clin. Trials **7**, 653–663 (2010)

Le Tourneau, C., Dieras, V., Tresca, P., Cacheux, W., Paoletti, X.: Current challenges for the early clinical development of anticancer drugs in the era of molecularly targeted agents. Target Oncol. **5**, 65–72 (2010)

Lin, Y., Shih, W.J.: Statistical properties of the traditional algorithm-based designs for phase I cancer clinical trials. Biostatistics **2**, 203–215 (2001)

Liu, S., Yuan, Y.: Bayesian optimal interval designs for phase I clinical trials. Appl. Stat. **64**, 507–523 (2015)

O'Quigley, J., Chevret, S.: Methods for dose finding studies in cancer clinical trials: a review. Stat. Med. **10**, 1647–1664 (1991)

O'Quigley, J., Pepe, M., Fisher, L.: Continual reassessment method: a practical design for phase I clinical trials in cancer. Biometrics **46**, 33–48 (1990)

Simon, R.M., Freidlin, B., Rubinstein, L., Arbuck, S.G., Collins, J., Chiristian, M.C.: Accelerated titration designs for phase I clinical trials in oncology. J. Natl. Cancer Inst. **89**, 1138–1147 (1997)

Skolnik, J.M., Barrett, J.S., Jayaraman, B., Patel, D., Adamson, P.C.: Shortening the timeline of pediatric phase I trials: the rolling six design. J. Clin. Oncol. **26**, 190–195 (2008)

Storer, B.E.: Design and analysis of phase I clinical trials. Biometrics **45**, 925–937 (1989)

Storer, B.E.: An evaluation of phase I clinical trial designs in the continuous dose-response setting. Stat. Med. **20**, 2399–2408 (2001)

Chapter 2
Dose Finding for a Combination of Two Agents

Abstract Two-agent combination trials—involving a dose combination of two already marketed drugs or a single new investigational drug to be used in combination with an approved drug—have rapidly increased in number. The concurrent development of two new agents intended for use in combination to treat a disease has attracted significant attention. Many authors have attempted to capture a dose–toxicity relationship for combination of two agents and to identify MTD combinations for two agents. This chapter reviews the dose-finding methods for two-agent combination trials along with the comparative analysis of these methods.

Keywords Combination of two agents · Comparative study · MTD combination Synergistic effect

2.1 Introduction

2.1.1 Two-Agent Combination Trials

The testing of drug combinations based on a strong biological rationale is increasingly seen in phase I trials. Effective treatment of cancer frequently requires the use of combinations of drugs because even if a cancer seems sensitive to one drug initially, cellular heterogeneity can lead to the emergence of drug-resistant disease (Marusyk et al. 2012). A combination of drugs can target cancer cells that have differing drug sensitivity levels, achieve a higher intensity of dose if the drugs have nonoverlapping toxicities, and can reduce the risk of drug resistance (Dancey and Chen 2006). Drug combinations have been repeatedly shown to improve survival among patients with either early-stage or advanced-stage cancer. Recently, cancer immunotherapies, such as monoclonal antibodies blocking the inhibitory programed cell death 1 pathway (PD-1–PD-L1), have made a great impact on cancer treatments. Despite the remarkable clinical efficacy of these agents against various malignant tumors, it was found that they are not sufficiently active for many patients. For example, to address this

© The Author(s), under exclusive licence to Springer Japan KK, part of Springer Nature 2018   9
A. Hirakawa et al., *Modern Dose-Finding Designs for Cancer Phase I Trials: Drug Combinations and Molecularly Targeted Agents*, JSS Research Series in Statistics, https://doi.org/10.1007/978-4-431-55573-5_2

issue, the combined inhibition of PD-1 and CTLA-4 in melanoma and non small cell lung cancer has highlighted the potential to further enhance the clinical benefits of monotherapies by combining agents with synergistic mechanisms of action (Kim and Alrwas 2014).

In the two-agent combination trials, estimation of the MTD combinations becomes more complex than for single-agent trials. When combining two agents, we need to consider a surface of probability of dose combinations where the dose of one or both agents can be altered. That is, multiple potential MTD combinations can be defined on the dose surface. The dose levels of two agents form various curves on the dose surface, called the MTD contour. We, therefore, need to precisely capture the dose–toxicity relationship for the combinations and to identify the MTD combination. Ideally, one or more MTD combinations should be identified while minimizing the total number of enrolled patients in phase I trials. Many authors have developed combination dose-finding methods, an overview of which is provided by Harrington et al. (2013). These methods can be generally classified as rule- or algorithm-based designs.

2.1.2   An Overview of Model-Based Dose-Finding Methods

In this chapter, we focus on model-based dose-finding methods for combinations, in which the primary aim is to find only *one* MTD combination. Conaway et al. (2004) estimated the MTD combination by determining the complete and partial orders of the toxicity probabilities by defining nodal and non-nodal parameters. A nodal parameter is one whose ordering is known with respect to all other parameters. Although the method of Conaway et al. (2004) does not rely on a parametric dose–toxicity model, it is not an algorithmic- or rule-based design; therefore, we chose to discuss it in the set of model-based approaches. This method was implemented in a phase I trial investigating induction therapy with bortezomib and vorinostat in patients with surgically resectable non small cell lung cancer (Jones et al. 2012). Yin and Yuan (2009a, b) developed Bayesian adaptive designs based on latent 2×2 tables and a copula-type model for two agents. Braun and Wang (2010) proposed a hierarchical Bayesian model for the probability of toxicity of two agents. Wages et al. (2011a, b) developed both Bayesian and likelihood-based designs that laid out possible complete orderings associated with the partial order and applied model selection techniques and the CRM to estimate the MTD combination. Hirakawa et al. (2013) proposed a dose-finding method based on the shrunken predictive probability of toxicity for combinations. Riviere et al. (2014) devised a Bayesian dose-finding design based on the logistic model, whereas Mander and Sweeting (2015) published a curve-free method that relies on the mathematical product of independent beta probabilities.

These methods can be roughly categorized into two groups: (1) those using a flexible model, with or without an interaction term, to jointly model the toxicity probability at each dose pair of the two agents; and (2) those that involve a more underparametrized approach, relying upon single-parameter "CRM-type" models and/or order-restricted inference (Barlow et al. 1972). For those in group (1), we focus on the method based on a copula-type (Yin and Yuan 2009b) model, termed the YYC method. We also introduce the method involving a hierarchical Bayesian model (Braun and Wang 2010), termed the BW method. Besides, we describe the methods using a shrinkage logistic model (Hirakawa et al. 2013), termed the HHM method, and the ordinary logistic model (Riviere et al. 2014), termed the RYDZ method. For the methods in group (2), we chose likelihood-based CRM for partial ordering (POCRM) (Wages et al. 2011b), termed the WCO method, as well as the order-restricted inference method of Conaway et al. (2004), termed the CDP method.

2.1.3 Methodological Characteristics

Here, we overview the six above-mentioned dose-finding methods. The methodological characteristics of each design are summarized in Table 2.1. The YYC, BW, and RYDZ methods have been developed based on Bayesian inference, whereas the HHM and WCO methods have been developed based on likelihood inference. The principle of CDP is the estimation procedure of Hwang and Peddada (1994). The YYC, HHM, and RYDZ methods model the interactive effect of two agents on the toxicity probability, but the BW method does not. The WCO method is based on the CRM and uses a class of underparametrized working models based on a set of possible orderings for the true toxicity probabilities. In terms of the restriction on skipping dose levels, the BW method allows for simultaneous escalation or de-escalation of both agents, whereas methods YYC, CDP, HHM, and RYDZ do not. Notably, the RYDZ method enables simultaneous escalation of both agents in the start-up dose escalation rule that is generally incorporated to gather enough information for Bayesian estimation at an early stage of trials. On the other hand, the WCO method allows for a flexible movement of dose levels throughout the trial and does not restrict movement to "neighbors" in the two-agent combination matrix.

In the following section, we introduce both the statistical model for capturing the dose–toxicity relationship and the dose-finding algorithm for exploring the MTD combinations because almost all the dose-finding methods for two-agent combination trials have often been developed by improving or devising these components of the method. The other detailed design characteristics are not shown in this book. We considered a two-agent combination trial using agents A_j ($j = 1, \ldots, J$) and B_k ($k = 1, \ldots, K$), respectively, throughout. We denote the probability of toxicity as π, and the targeting toxicity probability specified by physicians as ϕ. The other symbols are independently defined by the dose-finding methods we compared.

Table 2.1 Methodological characteristics of the six dose-finding methods. YYC = Yin and Yuan (2009b); CDP = Conaway, Dunbar, and Peddada (2004); BW = Braun and Wang (2010); WCO = Wages, Conaway, and O'Quigley (2011b); HHM = Hirakawa, Hamada, and Matsui (2013); RYDZ = Riviere, Yuan, Dubois, and Zohar (2014)

Method	YYC	CDP	BW	WCO	HHM	RYDZ
Estimation	Bayesian	Hwang and Peddada (1994)	Bayesian	Likelihood	Likelihood	Bayesian
Parametric dose–toxicity model	Copula	None	Hierarchical	Power	Shrinkage	Logistic
Prior toxicity probability specification	Yes	No	Yes	Yes	No	Yes
Inclusion of the interactive effect in the model	Yes	No	No	No	Yes	Yes
Cohort size used in the original paper	3	1	1	1	3	3
Restriction skipping on dose levels	One dose level of change only and not allowing simultaneous escalation or de-escalation of both agents	Same as the YYC method	One dose level of change only but allowing simultaneous escalation or de-escalation of both agents	No skipping restriction	Same as the YYC method	Same as the YYC method

2.2 The Bayesian Approach Based on Copula Regression

2.2.1 Copula-Type Models

Let p_j and q_k be the prespecified toxicity probability corresponding to A_j and B_k, respectively, and subsequently p_j^α and q_k^β will be the true probabilities of toxicity for agents A and B, respectively, where $\alpha > 0$ and $\beta > 0$ are unknown parameters. Let the true probability of toxicity at combination (A_j, B_k) be denoted as π_{jk}. Yin and Yuan (2009b) proposed to use a copula-type regression model in the form of

$$\pi_{jk} = 1 - \left\{ (1 - p_j^\alpha)^{-\gamma} + (1 - q_k^\beta)^{-\gamma} - 1 \right\}^{-1/\gamma}, \qquad (2.1)$$

where $\gamma > 0$ characterizes the interaction of two agents. They also introduced the use of the Gumbel–Hougaard copula model. The joint probability is modeled by

$$\pi_{jk} = 1 - \exp\left(-\left[\{-\log(1 - p_j^\alpha)\}^{1/\gamma} + \{-\log(1 - q_k^\beta)\}^{1/\gamma} \right]^\gamma \right). \qquad (2.2)$$

It should be noted that Gasparini et al. (2010) objected to the use of copulas for modeling the joint probability of toxicity because the above model has limitations in the modeling of drug–drug interactions. Further discussions are given in Gasparini et al. (2010).

For the method based on the copula model, using the data obtained at that time point, the posterior distribution is obtained by

$$f(\alpha, \beta, \gamma | \text{Data}) \propto L(\alpha, \beta, \gamma | \text{Data}) f(\alpha) f(\beta) f(\gamma), \qquad (2.3)$$

where $L(\alpha, \beta, \gamma | \text{Data})$ is the likelihood function of the model and $f(\alpha)$, $f(\beta)$, and $f(\gamma)$ are prior distributions, respectively. The Gibbs sampling algorithm is used to sample from the posterior distributions of the unknown parameters. When performing this procedure, we need to elicit the prior toxicity probabilities p_j and q_k from investigators. In two-agent combination phase I trials, the highest dose level of each agent may often be the MTD that has been identified in each monotherapy phase I trial; therefore, it is reasonable to set the prior toxicity probability of p_J (or q_K) equal to target ϕ (i.e., 0.30). The remaining toxicity probabilities $(p_1, \ldots, p_{J-1}$ and $q_1, \ldots, p_{K-1})$ could be based on the investigator elicitations, but it recommends selecting an even distribution from 0 to ϕ. We also need to specify hyperparameters α, β, and γ. Although we cannot change them in the software released by Yin and Yuan (2009b), those authors have examined the sensitivity of operating characteristics for α and β and reported that this method is robust at different hyperparameter values. The Gamma(2, 2) priors for α and β as well as the Gamma(0.1, 0.1) prior for γ are further recommended for the Clayton-type copula.

2.2.2 The Dose-Finding Algorithm

Suppose c_e and c_d are the fixed probability cutoffs for dose escalation and de-escalation, respectively. Dose escalation or de-escalation are restricted to one dose level of change only, while not allowing translation along the diagonal direction (corresponding to simultaneous escalation or de-escalation of both agents). As Yin and Yuan (2009b) pointed out in their paper, their dose-finding algorithm may be difficult to implement early in the trial owing to limited available data. Therefore, the following start-up rule is enforced to collect a certain amount of data for stabilizing parameter estimation before beginning the model-based dose finding.

1. Treat patients along the vertical dose escalation in the order $\{(A_1, B_1), \ldots, (A_1, B_K)\}$ until the first toxicity is observed.
2. Treat patients along the horizontal dose escalation in the order $\{(A_2, B_1), \ldots, (A_J, B_1)\}$ until the first toxicity is observed.

After the start-up rule for stabilizing parameter estimation, the dose-finding algorithm functions as follows:

1. If, at the current dose combination (j, k), $\Pr(\pi_{jk} < \phi) > c_e$, then the dose is escalated to an adjacent dose combination with the probability of toxicity higher than the current value and closest to ϕ. If the current dose combination is (A_J, B_K), then the doses remain at the same levels.
2. If, at the current dose combination (j, k), $\Pr(\pi_{jk} > \phi) > c_d$, then the dose is de-escalated to an adjacent dose combination with the probability of toxicity lower than the current value and closest to ϕ. In the case the current dose combination is (A_1, B_1), the trial is terminated.
3. Otherwise, the next cohort of patients continues to be treated with the current dose combination (doses staying at the same levels).
4. Once the maximum sample size $N_{\max}$ is achieved, the dose combination that has the probability of toxicity that is the closest to ϕ is selected as the MTD combination.

2.2.3 Software Implementation

In this section, we use the software released by Yin and Yuan (2009b) to implement their method. Readers can download the .exe file from

http://odin.mdacc.tmc.edu/~yyuan/index_code.html.

In this program, we input the following configurations: the number of dose levels for two agents, their true joint toxicity probabilities for dose combinations, the target toxicity probability, prior estimates of toxicity probabilities for dose levels for each agent, the total number of cohorts, the cohort size, and the number of simulated trials.

For example, we obtain the following simulation results when two dose levels for each agent are tested:

```
-------------------------------------------------
CPU time (hour)= 0.00208444      # of trials = 10
The number of cohorts = 10; cohort size = 3
Escalate if Pr(toxicity<0.3) > 0.8
De-escalate if Pr(toxicity<0.3) < 0.45

True toxicity probabilities:
   0.15    0.20    0.40
   0.10    0.15    0.35
   0.05    0.10    0.30

Selection probabilities (%):
  10.0    20.0    20.0
   0.0    20.0    10.0
   0.0     0.0    20.0

Number of patients treated at each dose:
   2.4     3.3     1.8
   3.3     1.2     2.4
   6.9     4.2     4.5

Number of toxicities observed at each dose:
   0.2     0.7     0.9
   0.5     0.5     0.9
   0.3     0.4     1.3

Total number of observed toxicities: 5.7
Percentage of inconclusive trials: 0.0%
-------------------------------------------------
```

At the default settings, c_e and c_d are set to 0.8 and 0.45, respectively. By means of the C++ program (copula.cpp), we can change the values for c_e and c_d. We can next select a copula model (i.e., Clayton or Gumbel copula model) and the prior distributions for their model parameters.

2.3 Hierarchical Bayesian Design

2.3.1 Hierarchical Models

Braun and Wang (2010) developed a novel hierarchical Bayesian design for combination trials. Let a_j and b_k be the dose levels corresponding to A_j and B_k, respectively, whose values are not the actual clinical values of the doses, but are the "effective" dose values that will lend stability to their dose–toxicity model. It is assumed that each π_{jk} has a beta distribution with parameters α_{jk} and β_{jk}. Notably, $\alpha_{jk}(\beta_{jk})$ can be interpreted as the prior number of patients assigned to combination (j, k) expected to manifest (or not manifest) toxicity. Braun and Wang (2010) proposed model α_{jk} and β_{jk} using the parametric functions of a_j and b_k,

$$\log\{\alpha_{jk}(\boldsymbol{\theta})\} = \theta_0 + \theta_1 a_j + \theta_2 b_k \quad \text{and} \quad \log\{\beta_{jk}(\boldsymbol{\lambda})\} = \lambda_0 - \lambda_1 a_j - \lambda_2 b_k, \quad (2.4)$$

respectively, where $\boldsymbol{\theta} = \{\theta_0, \theta_1, \theta_2\}$ obeys a multivariate normal distribution with mean $\boldsymbol{\mu} = \{\mu_0, \mu_1, \mu_2\}$, $\boldsymbol{\lambda} = \{\lambda_0, \lambda_1, \lambda_2\}$ follows a multivariate normal distribution with mean $\boldsymbol{\omega} = \{\omega_0, \omega_1, \omega_2\}$, and both $\boldsymbol{\theta}$ and $\boldsymbol{\lambda}$ have variance $\sigma^2 I_3$, in which I_3 is a 3 $\times$ 3 identity matrix. The samples from the posterior distribution for $(\boldsymbol{\theta}, \boldsymbol{\lambda})$ are easily obtained by Markov chain Monte Carlo methods. These samples lead to posterior distributions for each element of $\boldsymbol{\theta}$ and $\boldsymbol{\lambda}$, which in turn lead to a posterior distribution for each π_{jk}. The corresponding posterior means $\bar{\pi}_{jk}$ are calculated.

The BW method necessitates careful elicitation of priors and effective dose values. Development of priors begins with the specification of p_{j1} and q_{1k}, which are a priori values for $E(\pi_{j1})$ and $E(\pi_{1k})$. Braun and Wang (2010) set the lowest dose of each agent to zero, i.e., $a_1 = b_1 = 0$. Consequently, $\log(\alpha_{11}) = \theta_0$ and $\log(\beta_{11}) = \lambda_0$, and therefore θ_0 and λ_0 describe the expected number of toxicities for combination (A_1, B_1), and the remaining parameters in $\boldsymbol{\theta}$ and $\boldsymbol{\lambda}$ will describe how the expected toxicities for other combinations are related to (A_1, B_1). They also used the fact that

$$\frac{S p_{11}}{S(1 - p_{11})} = \frac{\alpha_{11}}{\beta_{11}} = \frac{\exp\{\theta_0\}}{\exp\{\phi_0\}} = \frac{\exp\{\mu_0\}}{\exp\{\omega_0\}}. \quad (2.5)$$

Then, the prior values for μ_0 and ω_0 are obtained via

$$\mu_0 = \log(S p_{11}) \quad \text{and} \quad \omega_0 = \log(S[1 - p_{11}]), \quad (2.6)$$

where $S = 1,000$ was chosen as a scaling factor to keep both hyperparameters sufficiently above 0. Furthermore, they select $\mu_1 = \mu_2 = \omega_1 = \omega_2 = 2\sqrt{\sigma^2}$ so that 97.5% of the prior distributions for $\theta_1, \theta_2, \lambda_1$, and λ_2 will lie above 0, depending upon the value of σ^2. Those authors point out that a value in the interval [5, 10] is often sufficient in their settings for adequate operating characteristics, but each trial setting will require fine-tuning of σ^2. They next define elicited odds ratios that can be approximated by

$$\tilde{\xi}_{j\cdot} \approx \exp\{(\mu_1 + \omega_1)a_j\} \quad \text{and} \quad \tilde{\xi}_{\cdot k} \approx \exp\{(\mu_2 + \omega_2)b_k\}, \quad (2.7)$$

in which effective doses are obtained by solving for a_j and b_k. All doses are rescaled to be proportional to log-odds ratios relative to combination (A_1, B_1). The derivation of priors and effective dose values in the BW method is somewhat complex, and it is recommended to read the original paper about the BW method for further detail.

We need to elicit the toxicity probability parameters p_{j1} and q_{1k} from investigators. As we described in the previous section, the values of p_{J1} and q_{1K} are generally set to 0.3, and the toxicity probabilities of all dose combinations are set arithmetically. We assessed operating characteristics of the BW method for three values of σ^2, i.e., $\sigma^2 = \{3, 5, 10\}$. The best overall performance was obtained with $\sigma^2 = 3$, while the BW method for $\sigma^2 = 5$ (or 10) performed worse in our simulations. This finding indicates that we need to fine-tune the value of σ^2 in practice, as Braun and Wang (2010) suggested.

2.3.2 The Dose-Finding Algorithm

The BW method accrues all patients in a single stage, rather than in two stages. The dose-finding algorithm is similar to that of the YYC method after the YYC start-up rule.

1. The first subject is assigned to combination (A_1, B_1).
2. Compute a 95% confidence interval for the overall toxicity rate among all combinations using the cumulative number of observed toxicities for subjects $1, 2, \ldots, (i-1)$. If the lower bound of the confidence interval is greater than the target toxicity rate, ϕ, terminate the trial.
3. Otherwise, use the outcomes and assignments of subjects $1, 2, \ldots, (i-1)$ to determine the posterior distribution of each π_{jk}, with posterior means $\bar{\pi}_{jk}$.
4. Extract the set of dose combinations, that is,

$$S = \{(j, k) \mid j_{i-1} - 1 \leq j \leq j_{i-1} + 1, k_{i-1} - 1 \leq k \leq k_{i-1} + 1\},$$

   that contains combinations that are within one dose level of the corresponding doses in the combination assigned to the most recently enrolled patient $(1, 2, \cdots, (i-1))$, and subsequently allocate the dose combination (j^*, k^*) in S as the one with the smallest $|\bar{\pi}_{jk} - \phi|$ to the next patient i.
5. Repeat these steps until maximum sample size $N_{\max}$ is reached. Upon completion of enrollment and follow-up of N_{max} patients, identify the MTD combination based on steps 3 and 4.

2.3.3 Software Implementation

To employ the BW method, readers can use the R code released at

http://www-personal.umich.edu/~tombraun/BraunWang/.

Brawn and Wang (2010) provided the following five pieces of code.

get.mtc.r   R code that will identify the optimal combination for the next patient to be enrolled based on the data collected on enrolled patients

run.onesim.r   R code that will run one simulated trial

jags model.txt   text file containing hierarchical model description in WinBUGS syntax

Actual Trial.r   R code to find a dose combination to assign to the fourth subject in a hypothetical trial

Simulation Study.r   Sample R code to run a simulation study composed of 1,000 simulations

The simulation study of the BW method can be easily executed by means of the run.onesim.r and jagsmodel.txt. We specify prior toxicity probabilities for each combination, true toxicity probabilities, the target rate of toxicity, maximum sample size, the prior variance parameter, starting doses, and the number of simulations. It should be noted that based on the results of our simulation studies, we recommend that the variance parameter σ^2 be set to 3 to stabilize the implementation of the R package **rjags**.

For example, the following simulation results are obtained if we execute the pieces of code below:

```
---------------------------------------------------
#Prior toxicity probabilities for each combination
p.prior <-
matrix(c(0.15,0.20,0.25,0.30,0.30,0.35,0.40,0.45),
nrow=2, ncol=4, byrow=TRUE)
#True toxicity probabilities
p.true <-
matrix(c(0.05,0.10,0.20,0.30,0.10,0.20,0.30,0.40),
nrow=2, ncol=4, byrow=TRUE)
#Targeted rate of DLTs
p.star <- 0.3
#Maximum sample size
m <- 30
#Prior variance parameter
s2 <- 3
#Starting doses
j.start <- 1
k.start <- 1
Run simulations
mysims <- NULL
Nsim <- 10
for (i in 1:Nsim)
{
  set.seed(i)
temp <-
run.onesim(m, p.true, p.prior, p.star, s2, j.start, k.start,
dir) mysims <- rbind(mysims, temp)
```

```
}
#Tabulate number of times each combo chosen as MTC
ndose.a <- ncol(p.prior)
ndose.b <- nrow(p.prior)
a <- mysims[,1]
b <- mysims[,2]
mtc.table <- table(c(b, paste(rep(0:ndose.b, ndose.a+1))),
c(a, rep(0:ndose.a, rep(ndose.b+1,ndose.a+1))))-1
rm(a,b)
colnames(mtc.table) <- paste(rep("A",ndose.a+1), 0:ndose.a,
sep="")
rownames(mtc.table) <- paste(rep("B",ndose.b+1), 0:ndose.b,
sep="")

> mtc.table
      A0 A1 A2 A3 A4
  B0  0  0  0  0  0
  B1  0  1  2  3  1
  B2  0  1  0  2  0

#Tabulate average number of patients assigned to each combo
a <- mysims[,m:(2*m-1)+4]
b <- t(matrix(as.numeric(paste(rep(1:ndose.a,ndose.b),
rep(1:ndose.b, rep(ndose.a,ndose.b)), sep="")),
        nrow=ndose.a*ndose.b, ncol=nrow(a)))
a <- cbind(a,b)
b <- t(apply(a, 1, table)-1)
nsubj.table <-
matrix(apply(b, 2, mean), ncol=ndose.a, nrow=ndose.b, byrow=F)
rm(a,b)
colnames(nsubj.table) <- paste(rep("A",ndose.a), 1:ndose.a,
sep="")
rownames(nsubj.table) <- paste(rep("B",ndose.b), 1:ndose.b,
sep="")

> nsubj.table
    A1  A2  A3  A4
B1 4.0 5.4 6.3 2.9
B2 2.9 4.4 2.4 1.7
--------------------------------------------------
```

2.4   An Approach Using a Shrinkage Logistic Model

2.4.1   The Shrinkage Logistic Model

Hirakawa et al. (2013) developed a dose-finding method based on the shrinkage logistic model. They first model the joint toxicity probability π_i for patient i using an ordinary logistic regression model with fixed intercept β_0 as follows:

$$\pi_i = \frac{\exp(\beta_0 + \beta_1 x_{i1} + \beta_2 x_{i2} + \beta_3 x_{i3})}{1 + \exp(\beta_0 + \beta_1 x_{i1} + \beta_2 x_{i2} + \beta_3 x_{i3})}, \tag{2.8}$$

where x_{i1} and x_{i2} are the actual (or standardized) dose levels of agents A and B, respectively, and x_{i3} represents a variable of their interaction such that $x_{i3} = x_{i1} \times x_{i2}$ for patient i.

Using the maximum likelihood estimates for parameters $\hat{\beta}_j$ ($j = 1, 2, 3$), Hirakawa et al. (2013) proposed the shrunken predictive probability:

$$\tilde{\pi}_i = \frac{\exp(\beta_0 + (1 - \delta_1)\hat{\beta}_1 x_{i1} + (1 - \delta_2)\hat{\beta}_2 x_{i2} + (1 - \delta_3)\hat{\beta}_3 x_{i3})}{1 + \exp(\beta_0 + (1 - \delta_1)\hat{\beta}_1 x_{i1} + (1 - \delta_2)\hat{\beta}_2 x_{i2} + (1 - \delta_3)\hat{\beta}_3 x_{i3})}, \tag{2.9}$$

where shrinkage multiplier $1 - \delta_j$ ($j = 1, 2$, and 3) is a number between 0 and 1. Hirakawa et al. (2013) also developed the method for estimation of the shrinkage multipliers.

2.4.2   The Dose-Finding Algorithm

Hirakawa et al. (2013) invoke the following start-up rule-based dose allocation algorithm with the cohort size of three until the maximum likelihood estimate for each parameter is obtained.

1. The matrix of combinations is zoned according to its diagonals from the upper left entry to the lower right entry, as described in the WCO method.
2. The first cohort is allocated to the zone that includes the lowest dose combinations (A_1, B_1). If a prespecified stopping rule is fulfilled, then we terminate the trial for safety. Otherwise, we will escalate to the next zone. If more than one dose combination is contained within a particular zone, we can sample without replacement from the dose combinations available, allocating the sampled dose combination to the next cohort. This sampling and allocation step is continued until all available dose combinations in that zone are tested.
3. During the above-mentioned step, the existence of maximum likelihood estimates for the regression coefficients is verified for every cohort of three patients, although we do not show this procedure in detail in this book. If we obtain the

maximum likelihood estimates, then the shrunken predictive probability of toxicity for each dose combination is calculated, and subsequently the following
dose-finding algorithm is applied.

After obtaining the maximum likelihood estimates for the regression parameters, we
calculate the shrunken predictive probability of toxicity for the current dose combination d_c and then start the following dose-finding algorithm. We adopt the same
restriction on the skipping dose level proposed in the YYC method. Let c_1 and c_2 be
the allowable bands from target toxicity limit ϕ as MTD combinations.

1. If, at the current dose combination d_c, $\phi - c_1 \leq \tilde{p}(d_c) \leq \phi + c_2$, then the next
   cohort of patients continues to be allocated to the current dose combination.
2. Otherwise, the next cohort of patients is allocated to the dose combination with
   the shrunken predictive probability closest to ϕ among the adjacent or current
   dose combinations.
3. Once the maximum sample size N_{max} is reached, the dose combination that should
   be assigned to the next cohort is selected as the MTD combination. In addition, if
   we encounter the situation where $d_c = d_1$ and $\tilde{p}(d_c) > \phi + c_2$, then we terminate
   the trial for safety.

2.4.3 Software Implementation

The estimation of shrinkage multipliers is carried out using the SAS/IML software
(SAS Institute Inc., Cart, NC). Given the data on dose levels of agents A and B, fixed
intercept (β_0), a maximum likelihood estimate for each coefficient ($\hat{\beta}_1$, $\hat{\beta}_2$, and $\hat{\beta}_3$),
and first-order linear approximation of π_i obtained by means of Eqs. (7) and (8) in
Hirakawa et al. (2013), we estimate the shrinkage parameters (δ_1, δ_2, and δ_3,) using
the following function module and the NLPNRR subroutine for the Newton–Raphson
ridge method in SAS/IML.

```
---------------------------------------------------
/************************************************/
d: shrinkage multipliers
dA: dose level of agent A
dB: dose level of agent B
Int: Fixed intercept
b1, b2, b3: Maximum likelihood estimate for each coefficient
pt: first-order linear approximation of true toxicity
    probability obtained using Equations (7) and (8)
    in ref. (Hirakawa et al., 20113)
/************************************************/

start l(d) global(dA,dB,Int, b1,b2,b3,pt);
```

```
ptilde=exp(Int+(1-d[1])#b1#dA+(1-d[2])#b2#dB
+(1-d[3])#b3#dA#dB)/(1+exp(Int+(1-d[1])#b1#dA
+(1-d[2])#b2#dB+(1-d[3])#b3#dA#dB));
logl=sum(pt#log(ptilde)+(1-pt)#log(1-ptilde));
return(logl);
finish l;

x0={0 0 0};
con={0 0 0,1 1 1};
optn={1 0};
call nlpnrr(rc,xr,"l",x0,optn,con);
if rc>0 then  d=xr[,1]||xr[,2]||xr[,3];
else  d=0||0||0;
```

2.5   An Approach Using a Logistic Model

2.5.1   The Logistic Model Involving Standardized Doses

Riviere et al. (2014) modeled the true probability of toxicity at combination (A_j, B_k) π_{jk} via an ordinary four-parameter logistic model as follows:

$$\text{logit}(\pi_{jk}) = \beta_0 + \beta_1 u_j + \beta_2 v_k + \beta_3 u_j v_k, \qquad (2.10)$$

where u_j and v_k are the standardized doses for the jth level of agent A and the kth level of agent B; $\beta_0, \beta_1, \beta_2$, and β_3 are unknown parameters that represent the intercept, the toxicity effects of agents A and B, and the interaction between the two agents, respectively. The standardized dose of two agents is defined as

$$u_j = \log\left(\frac{p_j}{1-p_j}\right), v_k = \log\left(\frac{q_k}{1-q_k}\right), \qquad (2.11)$$

where p_j and q_k are the prior probabilities of toxicity for agents A and B, respectively. Riviere et al. (2014) assumed a normal prior with mean 0 and variance 10 for the parameters of intercept (β_0) and interaction term (β_3), and presumed an exponential prior with a mean of 1 for β_1 and β_2. Thus, the joint posterior distribution of parameters $\beta_0, \beta_1, \beta_2$, and β_3 is given by

$$f(\beta_0, \beta_1, \beta_2, \beta_3 \mid \text{Data}) \propto L(\beta_0, \beta_1, \beta_2, \beta_3 \mid \text{Data}) f(\beta_0) f(\beta_1) f(\beta_2) f(\beta_3), \qquad (2.12)$$

where $L(\cdot)$ is the likelihood function of model parameters. The posterior samples for each parameter are obtained by the Gibbs sampler.

2.5.2   The Dose-Finding Algorithm

Riviere et al. (2014) applied the dose-finding algorithm proposed by Yin and Yuan (2009a). That is, they restricted dose escalation and de-escalation to one level at a time (i.e., we do not allow a dose to escalate or de-escalate along the diagonal). On the other hand, Sweeting and Mander (2012) showed that the diagonal escalation strategy may be more effective in reaching the target toxicity level with a limited sample size and can provide a higher percentage of correct selection of an MTD combination. They, therefore, adopted this strategy in their start-up rule of the RYDZ method. Notably, they also proposed a different criterion for the selection of an MTD combination at the end of the trial. Once trial reaches the maximum sample size, the RYDZ method selects the dose combination with the highest posterior probability,

$$Pr(\pi_{jk} \in [\phi - \delta, \phi + \delta]), \tag{2.13}$$

which has been used to treat at least one cohort of patients, as the MTD combination. Riviere et al. (2014) used δ of 0.1 in their simulation studies.

2.5.3   Software Implementation

We can avail ourselves of the RYDZ method using the R package **dfcomb**. Given the number and prior toxicity probabilities of agents A and B; values of ϕ, $\phi - \delta$, and $\phi + \delta$; the number of cohorts and cohort sizes; the probability threshold for dose escalation; dose de-escalation; and early trial termination with the minimum number of patients for early trial termination, the function **CombIncrease_sim** provides the operating characteristics of the RYDZ method as follows:

```
---------------------------------------------------
p_tox_sc1 = matrix(c(
0.10,0.20,0.30,
0.20,0.30,0.40,
0.30,0.40,0.50),nrow=3,ncol=3)
prior_a1 = c(0.1, 0.2, 0.3)
prior_a2 = c(0.1, 0.2, 0.3)
ndose_a1 = 3
ndose_a2 = 3

CombIncrease_sim(ndose_a1=ndose_a1, ndose_a2=ndose_a2,
p_tox=p_tox_sc1, target=0.30, target_min=0.20, target_max=0.40,
prior_tox_a1=prior_a1, prior_tox_a2=prior_a2, n_cohort=10,
cohort=3, tite=FALSE, nsim=1000, c_e=0.85, c_d=0.45, c_stop=1,
n_min=30, seed = 14061991)

True toxicities:
```

```
          Agent 1
Agent 2   1    2    3
       3 0.3 0.4 0.5
       2 0.2 0.3 0.4
       1 0.1 0.2 0.3


Percentage of Selection:
          Agent 1
Agent 2    1     2     3
       3 10.0 12.3   3.4
       2 12.9 27.8  11.0
       1  1.5 11.3   9.8


Number of patients:
          Agent 1
Agent 2   1     2     3
       3 1.99 2.38 2.14
       2 3.31 7.25 2.11
       1 5.81 2.92 2.10


Number of toxicities:
          Agent 1
Agent 2   1     2     3
       3 0.60 0.94 1.06
       2 0.65 2.15 0.87
       1 0.57 0.61 0.62


Percentage of inconclusive trials:  0
The minimum number of cohorts to stop the trial is:  10


Number of simulations:   1000
Cohort size:      3
Number of cohorts planned:   10
Total patients accrued:  30
Toxicity target:     0.3
Targeted toxicity interval:  [ 0.2 , 0.4 ]
Prior toxicity probabilities for agent 1:
[1] 0.1 0.2 0.3
Prior toxicity probabilities for agent 2:
[1] 0.1 0.2 0.3
Escalation threshold:    0.85
Deescalation threshold:  0.45
Stopping threshold:  1
Toxicity is not a time-to-event but binary
--------------------------------------------------
```

2.6 The Design Based on Order-Restricted Inference

2.6.1 Order-Restricted Inference

The method proposed by Conaway et al. (2004) is based on the estimation procedure of Hwang and Peddada (1994). Parameter estimation subject to order restrictions is discussed by Hwang and Peddada (1994) and Dunbar et al. (2001). The method of Hwang and Peddada (1994) uses different estimation procedures for "nodal" and "non-nodal" parameters. A nodal parameter is one whose ordering is known with respect to all the other parameters. For example, in a $J \times K$ matrix of drug combinations, the probability of toxicity, π_{11}, at combination (A_1, B_1) is a nodal parameter because it is known that $\pi_{11} \leq \pi_{j+1,k}$ and $\pi_{11} \leq \pi_{j,k+1}$ for $j, k \geq 1$. For nodal parameters, estimation proceeds by establishing a simple order that is consistent with the partial order. This is done by *guessing* the unknown inequalities and by obtaining isotonic regression estimates of nodal parameters π_{jk} based on the Pool Adjacent Violators Algorithm (PAVA). To estimate the non-nodal parameters, Hwang and Peddada (1994) eliminate the smallest number of parameters that make a non-nodal parameter into a nodal parameter. For instance, in a $J \times K$ matrix of drug combinations, π_{12} is a non-nodal parameter because it is unknown whether $\pi_{12} < \pi_{21}$ or vice versa. Estimates of the non-nodal parameters can be obtained in a version of PAVA for simple orders that fixes the nodal parameters at their previously estimated values. Hwang and Peddada (1994) demonstrated that the resulting estimates satisfy the partial order. Conaway et al. (2004) computed estimates of the parameters for all possible guesses and averaged them to eliminate the dependence of the estimates on a single guess in the ordering among non-nodal parameters.

The approach of Conaway et al.(2004) is a two-stage design. The initial stage is intended to quickly escalate through treatment combinations that are nontoxic (in single-patient cohorts until the first toxicity is observed), and the second stage implements the Hwang and Peddada (1994) approach. Throughout the second stage, the toxic response data for the ith treatment combination is of the form $Y = \{Y_{jk}; j = 1, \ldots, J; k = 1, \ldots, K\}$ with Y_{jk} equal to the number of observed toxicities among patients treated with combination (A_j, B_k). Suppose $\mathcal{A}$ denotes the set of treatments that have been administered thus far in the trial such that $\mathcal{A} = \{(j, k) : n_{jk} > 0\}$, where n_{jk} represents the number of patients treated with each combination. With the Beta(α_{jk}, β_{jk}) prior for π_{jk}, the toxicity probabilities are updated only for $(j, k) \in \mathcal{A}$.

$$\hat{\pi}_{jk} = \frac{Y_{jk} + \alpha_{jk}}{n_{jk} + \alpha_{jk} + \beta_{jk}} \tag{2.14}$$

The estimation procedure of Dunbar et al. (2001) is applied to the updated posterior means $\hat{\pi}_{jk}$ for $(j, k) \in \mathcal{A}$.

If appropriate prior information is available to investigators, it is described via a prior distribution of the form $\pi_{jk} \sim$ Beta(α_{jk}, β_{jk}). The investigators specify the expected value of π_{jk} and upper limit u_{jk} such that they are 95% certain that the toxicity probability will not exceed u_{jk}. The equations

$$E[\pi_{jk}] = \frac{\alpha_{jk}}{\alpha_{jk} + \beta_{jk}} \quad \text{and} \quad \Pr[\pi_{jk} \leq u_{jk}] = 0.95 \qquad (2.15)$$

are solved to obtain prior specifications for α_{jk} and β_{jk}. Another prior specification for the CDP method is to choose a subset of possible dose–toxicity orders based on ordering the combinations by rows, columns, and diagonals of the drug combination matrix. Following the guidance of Wages and Conaway (2013), we choose a subset of approximately 6–9 orderings. This approach provides an appropriate balance between choosing enough orderings so that we include adequate information to account for the uncertainty associated with partially ordered dose–toxicity curves, without increasing the dimensionality of the problem so much so that we diminish performance. We arrange orderings according to movements across rows, up columns, and along diagonals. Because in a large matrix, there could be many ways to arrange combinations along a diagonal, we restrict movements to only *moving across rows, up columns,* and *up or down any diagonal.*

2.6.2   The Dose-Finding Algorithm

Stage 1: The first patient is entered at the starting treatment, usually combination (A_1, B_1). The most appropriate treatment to which to escalate could possibly consist of more than one treatment combination. For example, in a matrix of combinations, the possible escalation treatment for $(1, 1)$ is $(1, 2)$ or $(2, 1)$. Therefore, if no toxicity is observed with $(1, 1)$, then the next patient is treated with a combination chosen from the "possible escalation treatments." If no toxicity is observed in this patient, the next patient is assigned to a combination randomly chosen from the set of possible escalation treatments that have not yet been administered in the trial. Once a toxicity is observed, Stage 2 begins.

Stage 2: For all $(j, k) \in \mathcal{A}$, we compute the loss, $L(\hat{\pi}_{jk}, \phi)$, associated with each combination. As in Conaway et al. (2004), we implement a symmetric loss function so that $L(\hat{\pi}_{jk}, \phi) = |\hat{\pi}_{jk} - \phi|$.

1. Suppose $l_{min} = \min_{(j,k)\in\mathcal{A}} L_{jk}(\hat{\pi}_{jk}, \phi)$, and let $\mathcal{C}$ be the set of combinations with losses equal to the minimum observed loss, $\mathcal{C} = \{(j, k) : L_{jk}(\hat{\pi}_{jk}, \phi) = l_{min}\}$.
2. If there is a single combination, $c \in \mathcal{C}$, then the suggested combination is c, with an estimated toxicity probability of $\hat{\pi}_c$
3. If $\mathcal{C}$ contains more than one combination, then we randomly choose among them according to the following rules:

   a. If $\hat{\pi}_c > \phi \,\forall\, c \in \mathcal{C}$, then we randomly choose from the set $\mathcal{C}$ of candidate combinations.

  b. If $\hat{\pi}_c \le \phi$ for at least one $c \in \mathcal{C}$, we choose randomly among the combina-
     tions in $\mathcal{C}$ that are expected to have the "highest" toxicity probability.

4. If the suggested combination has an estimated toxicity probability that is less
   than the target, a combination is chosen at random from the "possible escalation
   treatments" that have not yet been tested in the trial.

The averaged Hwang and Peddada (1994) estimates for each possible ordering pro-
duce estimates $\hat{\pi}_{jk}$ and the next patient is enrolled into the treatment with estimated
toxicity probability closest to the target rate such that $|\hat{\pi}_{jk} - \phi|$ is minimized. Sub-
sequent to a toxic or nontoxic response being observed for that patient, the toxicity
probabilities are re-estimated and the trial proceeds.

2.7   The Partial-Ordering Continual Reassessment Method

2.7.1   The Model for Possible Orderings of Toxicity Probability for a Dose Combination

The CRM for partial orders is based on utilizing a class of working models that correspond to possible orderings of the toxicity probabilities for the combinations. Specifically, suppose there are M possible orderings being considered that are indexed by
m. For a particular ordering, we model the true probability of toxicity, π_{jk}, corresponding to combination A_j and B_k, via a power model

$$\pi_{jk} \approx F_m(d_{jk}, \beta_m) = \left[p_{jk}(m) \right]^{\beta_m}; \quad m = 1, \ldots, M, \tag{2.16}$$

where $p_{jk}(m)$ represent the skeleton of the model at ordering m. We let the plausibility
of each ordering under consideration be described by a set of prior probabilities
$\tau = \{\tau(1), \ldots, \tau(M)\}$, where $\tau(m) \ge 0$ and $\sum \tau(m) = 1; m = 1, \ldots, M$. From
accumulated data Ω_i from i patients, the maximum likelihood estimate $\hat{\beta}_m$ of the
parameter β_m can be calculated for each of the m orderings, along with the value of
the log-likelihood, $\mathcal{L}_m(\hat{\beta}_m \mid \Omega_i)$, at $\hat{\beta}_m$. Wages et al. (2011b) proposed an escalation
method that first chooses the ordering that maximizes the updated probability

$$\omega(m) = \frac{\exp\{\mathcal{L}_m(\hat{\beta}_m \mid \Omega_i)\}\tau(m)}{\displaystyle\sum_{m=1}^{M} \exp\{\mathcal{L}_m(\hat{\beta}_m \mid \Omega_i)\}\tau(m)} \tag{2.17}$$

before inclusion of each patient. If we denote this ordering as m^*, they use estimate
$\hat{\beta}_{m^*}$ to evaluate the toxicity probabilities for each combination at ordering m^* so that
$\hat{\pi}_{jk} \approx F_{m^*}(d_{jk}, \hat{\beta}_{m^*})$.

A prior specification for the WCO method is to choose a subset of possible dose–toxicity orders. We rely on the guidance of Wages and Conaway (2013) and choose approximately 6–9 orderings based on ordering the combinations by rows, columns, and diagonals of the drug combination matrix. Another specification that needs to be made prior to beginning the study is a set of skeleton values $p_{jk}(m)$. We can rely on the algorithm of Lee and Cheung (2009) to generate reasonable skeleton values using function **getprior** in **R** package **dfcrm**. We simply need to specify skeleton values at each combination that is adequately spaced (O'Quigley and Zohar 2010) and to adjust them to correspond to each possible ordering, in order for the WCO method to show good performance in terms of identifying an MTD combination. The location of these skeleton values can be adjusted to correspond to each possible ordering using the **getwm** function in **R** package **pocrm** (Wages and Varhegyi 2013).

2.7.2 The Dose-Finding Algorithm

Within the framework of sequential likelihood estimation, an initial escalation scheme is needed, given that the likelihood fails to have a solution in the interior of the parameter space unless some heterogeneity (i.e., at least one toxic and one nontoxic) in the responses has been observed.

Stage 1: At the first stage, the WCO method makes use of "zoning" the matrix of combinations according to its diagonals. The trial begins in zone $Z_1 = \{(A_1, B_1)\}$, and the first cohort of patients is to be enrolled in this "lowest" combination. After the first detection of a toxicity in one of the patients, the first stage is closed, and the second (model-based) stage is opened. As long as no toxicities occur, cohorts of patients are examined at each dose within the currently occupied zone, before escalating to the next highest zone. If (A_1, B_1) was tried and deemed "safe," then the trial will escalate to zone $Z_2 = \{(A_1, B_2), (A_2, B_1)\}$. If more than one dose is present within a zone, we can sample without replacement from the doses available within the zone. Therefore, the next cohort is enrolled into a dose that is chosen randomly from (A_1, B_2) and (A_2, B_1). The trial is not allowed to advance to zone Z_3 at the first stage until a cohort of patients has been observed at all combinations in Z_2. This procedure continues until a toxicity is observed or all available zones are exhausted.

Stage 2: Subsequent to a toxicity being observed, the second stage of the trial begins.

1. Based on accumulated data Ω_i from i patients, the estimated toxicity probabilities $\hat{\pi}_{jk}$ are obtained for all combinations being tested, by the procedure described above.
2. The next entering patient is then allocated to the dose combination with the estimated toxicity probability closest to the target toxicity rate so that $|\hat{\pi}_{jk} - \phi|$ is minimized.

3. There is no skipping the restriction imposed on escalation to allow for adequate exploration of the drug combination space.
4. For trials subject to partial ordering, there may be more than one combination with toxicity probability closest to the target. If there is a "tie" between two or more combinations, the patient will be randomized to one of the combinations with the toxicity probability closest to the target. The trial stops once enough information accumulates about the MTD combination.

2.7.3 Software Implementation

Readers can apply the WCO method using R package **pocrm**. Given the true toxicity probabilities of agents A and B, the possible orderings, skeleton values, initial guesses of toxicity probabilities for each ordering based on function **getprior** in **R** package **dfcrm**, prior probability for each possible ordering, the size of patient cohorts, the number of patients for the stopping rule, maximum sample size, target toxicity rate, the number of simulations, and an acceptable toxicity range, function **pocrm.sim** provide the operating characteristics of the WCO method as follows:

```
--------------------------------------------------
#True toxicity rates .
r<-c(0.05,0.10,0.15,0.20,0.15,0.20,0.30,0.35,0.20
,0.30,0.60,0.70,0.60,0.65,0.70,0.80)
#Specify the possible orderings.
orders<-matrix(nrow=3,ncol=16)
orders[1,]<-c(1,2,5,3,6,9,4,7,10,13,8,11,14,12,15,16)
orders[2,]<-c(1,5,2,3,6,9,13,10,7,4,8,11,14,15,12,16)
orders[3,]<-c(1,5,2,9,6,3,13,10,7,4,14,11,8,15,12,16)
#Specify the skeleton values.
skeleton<-c(0.20,0.22,0.24,0.26,0.28,0.30,0.32,
0.34,0.36,0.38,0.40,0.42,0.44,0.46,0.48,0.50)
#Initial guesses of toxicity probabilities for each ordering.
alpha<-getwm(orders,skeleton)
#We consider all orders to be equally likely prior to the study.
prior.o<-rep(1/3,3)
#Initial escalation at Stage 1 proceeds according to the zones.
#Single patient cohorts are used.
x0<-c(rep(1,1),rep(2,1),rep(5,1),rep(3,1),rep(6,1),
rep(9,1),rep(4,1),rep(7,1),rep(10,1),rep(13,1),
rep(8,1),rep(11,1),rep(14,1),rep(12,1),rep(15,1),rep(16,1))
#Number of patients used to define stopping rule
stop<-31
#Maximum sample size.
```

```
n<-30
#The target toxicity rate
theta<-0.30
#Number of simulations
nsim<-100
#Definition of acceptable toxicity rates
tox.range<-0.05
fit<-pocrm.sim(r,alpha,prior.o,x0,stop,n,theta,nsim,tox.range)
fit
$true.prob
 [1] 0.05 0.10 0.15 0.20 0.15 0.20 0.30 0.35 0.20
 0.30 0.60 0.70 0.60 0.65 0.70 0.80
$MTD.selection
 [1] 0.00 0.00 0.07 0.20 0.01 0.08 0.19 0.03 0.10
 0.19 0.04 0.00 0.08 0.01 0.00 0.00
$patient.allocation
 [1] 0.07 0.06 0.07 0.11 0.05 0.09 0.12 0.04 0.09
 0.10 0.04 0.01 0.09 0.02 0.01 0.02
$percent.toxicity
[1] 0.3016667
$mean.n
[1] 30
$acceptable
[1] 0.41


---------------------------------------------------
```

2.8 Operating Characteristics

Little is known about the relative performance of competing model-based dose-finding methods for combination phase I trials. Some authors have compared their method with existing model-based methods (Wages et al. 2011a, b; Hirakawa et al. 2013). Wages et al. (2011b) reported that their method is competitive in comparison with the previously proposed method of Wages et al. (2011a), which has been demonstrated to have performance comparable to that of the methods of Conaway et al. (2004) and Yin and Yuan (2009a, b). Hirakawa et al. (2013) reported that their method is competitive relative to the methods of Yin and Yuan (2009a) and Wages et al. (2011b).

Riviere et al. (2014) compared two algorithm-based and four model-based dose-finding methods by means of three evaluation indices under 10 scenarios of a 3×5 dose combination matrix. Specifically, the two up-and-down designs using isotonic regression and the T-statistic proposed by Ivanova and Wang (2004) and Ivanova and Kim (2009), respectively, were selected as the algorithm-based methods; the logarithm, Clayton, and Gumbel model-based methods proposed by Wang and Ivanova (2005) and Yin and Yuan (2009a, b), respectively, as well as the partial-ordering CRM proposed by Wages and Conaway (2011a) were selected as model-based methods. Among their conclusions was that the model-based methods performed better than the algorithm-based ones, as demonstrated in single-agent studies (Iasonos et al. 2008).

These comparisons have been made at limited and ideal settings with respect to the type of combination matrix, the position, and number of true MTD combinations, using few evaluation indices, and often for large sample sizes (i.e., ~60). Nonetheless, in practice, we often encounter complex and various settings of phase I trials. Specifically, (1) the dose combination matrices are not only of the square type (i.e., 3×3 and 4×4) but also of the rectangle type (2×4 and 3×5); (2) the underlying position and number of true MTD combinations possibly vary; and (3) the sample size is as small as 30 in practice. Furthermore, the operating characteristics of the dose-finding methods developed based on different principles should be compared via many evaluation indices. Hirakawa et al. (2015) and Hirakawa and Sato (2016) examined performance of six methods based on six evaluation indices under 16 toxicity scenarios shown in Table 2.2. The target toxicity probability that is clinically allowed, ϕ, is set to 0.3. For each simulated trial, no stopping rule was specified to exhaust prespecified maximum sample size $N_{\max} = 30$. Each simulation study consisted of 1,000 trials. The other configurations of the methods are elaborated by Hirakawa et al. (2015) and Hirakawa and Sato (2016). The aim of simulation studies was to evaluate (1) how well each method identifies MTD combinations at and near the target rate, (2) how well each method allocates patients to combinations at and around the true MTD combination, and (3) how feasible it is to implement each method given its respective prior specifications and software capabilities.

Across the 16 scenarios, the YYC, CDP, BW, WCO, HHM, and RYDZ methods yielded average 34, 47, 40, 46, 42, and 48% recommendation rates for true MTD combinations, respectively. The YYC, CDP, BW, WCO, HHM, and RYDZ methods showed average 41, 30, 33, 32, 25, and 31% recommendation rates for overly toxic dose combinations, respectively. The average number of patients allocated to true MTD combinations of the YYC, CDP, BW, WCO, HHM, and RYDZ methods averages 6, 11, 9, 10, 8, and 9, respectively. The overall percentages of observed toxicities of methods YYC, CDP, BW, WCO, HHM, and RYDZ were averaged 23, 32, 30, 28, 20, and 27%, respectively. The average number of patients allocated to a dose combination above the true MTD combinations of the YYC, CDP, BW, WCO, HHM, and RYDZ methods averages 8, 12, 11, 9, 5, and 8, respectively. In considering a benchmark for this summary measure, Cheung (2011) analyzed the ideal situation in which all patients are treated with the true MTD combination. In this case, we would expect a $\phi = 30\%$ observed toxicity rate. Therefore, a design that results in roughly $\phi\%$ toxicities on average per trial can be regarded as safe. The CDP, BW, and WCO methods yield the best performance with respect to an observed toxicity rate closest to the target toxicity rate. Cheung (2011) also consider that the recommendation rates for true MTD combinations are the most immediate index for accuracy, which can be used to compare different methods, while the entire distri-

Table 2.2 Summary of the operating characteristics

Scenarios Methods	1	2	3	4	5	6	7	8	9	10	11	12	13	14	15	16	Average
Recommendation rates for true MTD combinations (%)																	
YYC	44	70	26	6	59	44	33	5	39	49	72	2	30	18	37	2	34
CDP	62	81	25	29	80	43	46	23	53	41	92	38	51	39	34	22	47
BW	50	66	24	36	58	37	28	24	39	38	83	29	38	33	33	20	40
WCO	56	73	32	31	77	40	37	23	49	48	86	36	39	44	41	26	46
HHM	45	66	28	38	64	49	31	29	47	46	70	22	30	44	42	20	42
RYDZ	48	85	30	50	82	50	33	42	35	35	84	40	34	57	35	24	48
Recommendation rates for overly toxic dose combinations (%)																	
YYC	23	23	54	70	27	32	42	55	26	40	n/a	47	25	41	49	54	41
CDP	24	18	54	36	10	41	20	39	10	34	n/a	25	26	37	47	32	30
BW	27	24	48	37	17	39	25	41	26	39	n/a	32	28	37	43	35	33
WCO	24	24	55	44	13	36	29	46	20	29	n/a	36	19	32	34	34	32
HHM	14	23	48	36	12	22	22	32	12	19	n/a	29	15	31	24	32	25
RYDZ	27	14	57	35	11	36	22	42	18	35	n/a	21	26	29	40	47	31
Average number of patients allocated to true MTD combinations																	
YYC	8	14	6	1	12	9	5	1	6	10	10	1	6	4	8	0	6
CDP	14	17	5	6	17	9	11	5	12	10	24	8	11	8	8	5	11
BW	11	14	5	9	12	8	6	6	10	8	23	5	8	8	6	4	9
WCO	14	16	7	7	16	10	7	5	11	12	21	8	8	10	9	5	10
HHM	11	14	6	6	9	8	3	5	8	9	15	5	5	7	7	3	8
RYDZ	11	15	4	10	14	10	5	8	8	7	20	7	6	12	5	3	9

(continued)

Table 2.2 (continued)

Scenarios

Methods	1	2	3	4	5	6	7	8	9	10	11	12	13	14	15	16	Average
Overall percentage of observed toxicities (%)																	
YYC	22	27	25	22	24	24	24	25	18	24	20	26	22	26	24	22	23
CDP	31	39	36	28	32	34	31	34	25	31	27	35	31	35	31	30	32
BW	30	34	32	29	31	31	29	31	27	31	27	33	31	32	30	30	30
WCO	28	35	33	27	26	27	23	28	25	29	26	32	26	28	26	24	28
HHM	22	33	28	19	15	18	15	19	17	24	21	29	18	20	17	13	20
RYDZ	27	31	29	26	28	26	25	26	24	27	24	28	26	28	26	29	27
Average number of patients allocated to a dose combination above the true MTD combinations																	
YYC	3	6	11	11	6	5	9	10	3	9	n/a	9	4	10	9	9	8
CDP	10	11	18	12	7	15	9	15	4	12	n/a	12	10	14	15	12	12
BW	9	10	15	11	8	12	9	12	8	12	n/a	12	10	13	14	12	11
WCO	7	9	16	11	4	9	6	12	5	9	n/a	11	6	9	9	8	9
HHM	3	11	14	7	0	3	3	6	2	6	n/a	9	1	5	3	2	5
RYDZ	7	8	14	8	6	7	7	8	4	10	n/a	7	7	8	10	13	8
Accuracy index																	
YYC	0.40	0.72	0.47	0.31	0.58	0.45	0.46	0.30	0.43	0.54	0.37	0.36	0.50	0.42	0.58	0.34	0.45
CDP	0.56	0.82	0.49	0.48	0.78	0.56	0.66	0.53	0.60	0.53	0.56	0.60	0.67	0.56	0.55	0.53	0.59
BW	0.37	0.71	0.47	0.49	0.55	0.49	0.46	0.51	0.42	0.39	0.40	0.54	0.50	0.45	0.48	0.47	0.48
WCO	0.46	0.76	0.58	0.50	0.74	0.53	0.60	0.51	0.55	0.59	0.47	0.64	0.61	0.57	0.58	0.53	0.57
HHM	0.31	0.69	0.49	0.54	0.62	0.62	0.56	0.58	0.54	0.52	0.37	0.56	0.48	0.56	0.50	0.40	0.52
RYDZ	0.36	0.86	0.56	0.65	0.78	0.61	0.59	0.66	0.56	0.49	0.44	0.67	0.57	0.66	0.51	0.45	0.59

bution of selected dose combinations does provide more detailed information than what the recommendation rates for true MTD combinations alone suggest. Cheung (2011) proposed the accuracy index, after n patients, defined as

$$M_n = 1 - J \times K \times \frac{\sum_{j=1}^{J} \sum_{k=1}^{K} |\pi_{jk} - \phi| \times \rho_{jk}}{\sum_{j=1}^{J} \sum_{k=1}^{K} |\pi_{jk} - \phi|}, \qquad (2.18)$$

where π_{jk} is the true toxicity probability of dose combination (A_j, B_k), and ρ_{jk} is the probability of selecting dose combination (A_j, B_k). A large index indicates high accuracy, and the maximum value of the index is 1. Based on the accuracy index, the CDP and RYDZ methods showed the maximum value, 0.59, and the WCO method showed the second largest value: 0.57.

2.9 Effects of Design Properties

Many model-based methods include four design properties: patient cohort size, dose–toxicity model, choice of the start-up rule, and whether or not to include a restriction on dose-level skipping. In the studies by Riviere et al. (2014) and Hirakawa et al. (2015), these design properties were kept as close as possible to those in published works, to be true to the original design intended by the authors because their goals were to compare the dose-finding designs implied by these published methods. Nevertheless, the rationale for choosing each design property, particularly the patient cohort size, dose–toxicity model, start-up rule, and whether or not to include a restriction on dose-level skipping, was not substantially investigated in these studies. When statisticians develop a new dose-finding method or modify an existing method, they are especially interested in the true effects of these properties. Thus, a fair comparison of these properties is necessary. Moreover, when planning phase I trials, investigators may need to change the four design properties of the model-based method for practical or ethical reasons. In such cases, understanding the true effects of these properties on the operating characteristics would be beneficial.

Hirakawa et al. (2016) analyzed the well-known four design properties and evaluated the impact of each independent effect on the operating characteristics of the dose-finding method at these properties. With respect to the properties of the design properties in the dose-finding methods for two-agent combination trials, Sweeting and Mander (2012) evaluated various dose escalation strategies in the six- and three-parameter dose–toxicity models for two-agent combination trials using a cohort size of two patients. Hirakawa et al. (2016) performed comprehensive simulation studies to primarily examine the effects of the four design properties on the identification of the true MTD combinations and exposure to unacceptable toxic dose combinations at the complex and various settings of two-agent combination trials.

In this section, we touch on the patient cohort size, the choice of a start-up rule, and whether or not to include a restriction on dose level skipping, along with the insights obtained from the results of the simulation studies (for examining the effects of these design properties) conducted by Hirakawa et al. (2016).

2.9.1 Size of Patient Cohorts

Dose-finding designs allocate a cohort of patients to each dose combination. The size of patient cohorts typically described in the statistical literature is conventionally in the range of 1–3 and may be related to the probability of identifying the true MTD combination. This is because the total number of doses that can be tested during the trial depends on the number of patients and the size of the cohort. Notably, we supposed that the total sample size is fixed, and only the distribution into cohorts is the design element. For example, for a total sample size of 30, a cohort size of 1, 2, or 3 results in the use of up to 30, 15, or 10 doses, respectively. In this example, the cohort size of 3 enables toxicity data to be collected from more patients for a given dose combination. On the other hand, the opportunity to explore more dose combinations is lost. Selecting an appropriate cohort size is therefore an important consideration for investigators when designing a phase I trial.

According to the results of the simulation studies conducted by Hirakawa et al. (2016), we observed that the selection rates for true MTD combinations decreased, and those for unacceptable toxicity dose combinations increased on average with the increasing patient cohort sizes. To have the best chance to identify the true MTD combination and to avoid unacceptable toxicity of dose combinations, a cohort size of 1 may be favorable and unrelated to any of the other design properties. We expect that at a cohort size of 1, the selection rates for true MTD combinations are up to 5% higher than in studies that involve a cohort size of 2 or 3. Nonetheless, the use of a cohort size of 1 may be controversial in some trials, owing to concerns about the determination of dose escalation or de-escalation based on toxicity data from only one patient, especially at an early stage of a trial. Therefore, the development of a dose-finding method with variable patient cohort sizes during the trial is necessary, as stated by Kakurai et al. (2015). In addition, the smaller cohort size operationally requires more time to complete the trials. Depending on the circumstances of trial operation, one may prefer a cohort size of 2 (or 3) in practice.

2.9.2 The Choice of a Dose–Toxicity Model

To accommodate synergistic toxicity effects in two-agent combinations, several useful models have been proposed. For example, Thall et al. (2003) published a six-parameter model for determining the toxicity probabilities of dose combinations and a toxicity equivalence contour for two-agent combinations. Wang and Ivanova (2004) proposed a logistic-type logarithm model. Yin and Yuan (2009a) introduced the use of the Clayton and Gumbel copula-type model. Hirakawa et al. (2013) developed a shrinkage logistic model with an interaction term of two agents. When selecting a dose–toxicity model, one should pay attention to the number of parameters included in the model because this characteristic affects the results at limited sample sizes. In the present study, we focused on well-known three-parameter models for the following reasons: First, over the last decade, many authors tended to propose a three-parameter model rather than a one- or six-parameter model. To this end, authors of recent comparative studies on the rival dose-finding methods chose the methods based on the three-parameter models as competitors (Riviere et al. 2014; Hirakawa et al. 2015). Second, in addition to the specification of the four design properties chosen in this study, the specifications of the partial orderings are required for the one-parameter model (Wages et al. 2011a, b). With respect to the partial orderings, a key assumption for dose-finding methods for single-agent trials is the monotonicity of the dose–toxicity curve. In this case, the curve is said to follow a "complete order" because the ordering of probabilities of toxicity for any pair of doses is known, and administration of greater doses of the agent can be expected to yield toxicity in an increasing proportion of patients. In studies testing combinations, the probabilities of toxicity often follow a partial order, in that there are pairs of combinations for which the ordering of the toxicity probabilities is not known. Such an assumption would make the comparison between the one-parameter and three-parameter models unsubstantial. Specifically, although we can compare the performance between the composite of one-parameter models and partial orderings and three-parameter models, we cannot fairly compare the independent (or crude) effects between the one-parameter and three-parameter models. Third, a fair comparison between the operating characteristics of the three-parameter and six-parameter models is also difficult because the six-parameter model described by Thall et al. (2003) also requires the inherent specifications of prior distributions for the model parameters. In the study by Hirakawa et al. (2016), the following logistic-type logarithm model introduced by Wang and Ivanova (2005) and modified by Gasparini (2013)—in addition to the Clayton and Gumbel Archimedean copula models proposed by Yin and Yuan (2009a)—were compared.

$$\text{Logarithm model} \quad \pi_{jk} = 1 - (1 - p_j)^\alpha (1 - q_k)^{\beta - \alpha\beta\gamma \log(1 - p_j)}, \qquad (2.19)$$

where π_{jk} is the joint toxicity probability when combining agent A_j ($j = 1, \ldots, J$) and B_k ($k = 1, \ldots, K$); p_j and q_k are the prespecified toxicity probabilities corresponding to agents A_j and B_k, respectively.

Simulation studies revealed that the results generated by the dose–toxicity model are independent of whether the dose combination matrix is square or rectangular and of the position of MTD combinations in the dose combination matrix. All three dose–toxicity models evaluated were similar on average. Although we thoroughly examined the operating characteristics of the three dose–toxicity models, there may be frequently encountered situations that we did not consider. For instance, our simulations implied that the two agents are already approved because the prior toxicity probabilities for the highest dose level of both agents were commonly set to 0.30. The highest dose level for each agent is assumed to be the MTD that has been determined in a single-agent trial. Thus, we assumed that the lowest and highest doses are both fixed in our simulation studies. In practice, however, phase I trials can involve combinations of new and approved agents or two new agents. Further simulation studies are necessary to optimize the dose-finding design for such trials. In addition to the specifications of prior toxicity probability, the operating characteristics of the dose–toxicity models vary depending on the prior distributions of model parameters in the dose combination matrix. Therefore, the reasonable choice of a dose–toxicity model may be the most difficult issue in planning dose-finding trials.

2.9.3 The Start-Up Rule

The start-up dose allocation rule is a rule-based algorithm that is applied until a certain amount of data is obtained. This rule is generally introduced to stabilize the Bayesian estimation of parameters in a chosen dose–toxicity model. For example, the start-up rule is often applied until toxicity is first observed. Here, we introduced the two popular start-up rules: those proposed by Yin and Yuan (2009a) and by Wages et al. (2011b). The start-up rule proposed by Yin and Yuan (2009a) involves treating patients along the vertical dose escalation in the order $(A_1, B_1), (A_1, B_2), \cdots$ until the first dose-limiting toxicity (toxicity) is observed. Patients are then treated along the horizontal dose escalation in the order $(A_2, B_1), (A_3, B_1), \cdots$ until the first toxicity is observed. We refer to this as the vertical and horizontal (VH) rule. A model-based dose-finding method is then designed. The rule of Wages et al. (2011b) begins with dividing the dose combination matrix into several groups along the diagonals of the combination matrix. For example, in a 4×4 dose combination matrix, seven groups are generated. The trial begins at the lowest combination (A_1, B_1) (the first group) and, in the absence of toxicity, escalates to the second group, (A_1, B_2) and (A_2, B_1). At this step, if the second cohort is allocated to (A_1, B_2), we then automatically allocate the third cohort to (A_2, B_1) and vice versa. That is, we sample without replacement from the dose combinations available until all the available dose combinations in that group are tested as long as no toxicity occurs. We refer to this principle as the diagonal rule.

In simulation studies, the VH and diagonal start-up rules may result in similar average selection rates for true MTD combinations and unacceptable toxicity dose combinations, irrespective of the dose combination matrix and MTD combination position. In addition, the VH rule is operationally easier to apply than the diagonal rule because it does not include a random sampling procedure.

2.9.4 Restrictions on Skipping Dose Levels

Any restrictions imposed on the skipping of dose levels during model-based dose finding may be a controversial issue in many phase I trials because of safety concerns.

The original CRM proposed by O'Quigley et al. (1990) allows us to skip dose levels during dose escalation or de-escalation in single-agent phase I trials. Partial-ordering CRM for identifying MTD combinations in two-agent combination phase I trials also imposes no restriction on dose-level skipping. Nevertheless, several authors argued that moving from a given dose, (A_j, B_k), to dose (A_{j+1}, B_{k+1}) (i.e., increasing the doses of both agents) may expose patients to a higher risk of toxicity (Yin and Yuan, 2009a; Wages et al. 2011b). Therefore, it has been proposed that dose escalation or de-escalation should be restricted such that doses change only by one level at a time, and that the doses of both drugs are never simultaneously increased or simultaneously decreased (Restriction 1). The allowed dose combinations of Restriction 1 are defined as the following set:

$$S_1 = \{(j-1,k), (j+1,k), (j,k), (j,k+1), (j,k-1), (j+1,k-1), (j-1,k+1)\}. \tag{2.20}$$

Although Braun and Wang (2010) also limit dose adjustment to one level of change only, they allow simultaneous escalation or de-escalation of both agents (Restriction 2). Restriction 2 is defined by the following set:

$$\begin{aligned} S_2 = \{&(j-1,k), (j+1,k), (j,k), (j,k+1), (j,k-1), (j+1,k-1), \tag{2.21}\\ &(j-1,k+1), (j-1,k-1), (j+1,k+1)\} \end{aligned}$$

Investigators should decide which type of restriction to use based on historical toxicity data of combinations of the two agents. Ultimately, for two drugs that are already approved, there will be more toxicity data available, and dose skipping can likely be less restricted.

In simulation studies, restricting dose-level skipping may improve the selection rates of true MTD combinations by up to 10% and could reduce the selection rates of dose combinations with unacceptable toxicity by up to 4% in our simulation studies. Nonetheless, the effect of restriction on skipping a dose level varied depending on the patient cohort size. We recommend including a restriction on skipping dose levels when the cohort size is greater than or equal to 2. The choice of Restriction 1 or Restriction 2 makes no difference and, therefore, the choice can be conveniently made in many cases. To alleviate concerns regarding simultaneous escalation of the two agents during the trial, Restriction 1 may be appealing in practice.

References

Barlow, R.E., Bartholomew, D.J., Bremner, J.M., Brunk, H.D.: Statistical Inference under Order Restrictions: Theory and Application of Isotonic Regression. Wiley, London (1972)

Braun, T.M., Wang, S.: A hierarchical Bayesian design for phase I trials of novel combinations of cancer therapeutic agents. Biometrics **66**, 805–812 (2010)

Cheung, Y.K.: Dose Finding by the Continual Reassessment Method. Chapman and Hall, London (2011)

Conaway, M.R., Dunbar, S., Peddada, S.D.: Designs for single- or multiple-agent phase I trials. Biometrics **60**, 661–669 (2004)

Dancey, J.E., Chen, H.X.: Strategies for optimizing combinations of molecularly targeted anticancer agents. Nat. Rev. Drug Discov. **5**, 649–659 (2006)

Dunbar, S., Conaway, M.R., Peddada, S.D.: On improved estimation of parameters subject to order restrictions. Stat. Appl. **3**, 121–128 (2001)

Gasparini, M.: General classes of multiple binary regression models in dose finding problems for combination therapies. Appl. Stat. **62**, 115–133 (2013)

Gasparini, M., Bailey, S., Neuenschwander, B.: Correspondence: Bayesian dose finding in oncology for drug combinations by copula regression. Appl. Stat. **59**, 543–544 (2010)

Harrington, J.A., Wheeler, G.M., Sweeting, M.J., Mander, A.P., Jodrell, D.I.: Adaptive designs for dual-agent phase I dose-escalation studies. Nat. Rev. Clin. Oncol. **10**, 277–288 (2013)

Hirakawa, A., Hamada, C., Matsui, S.: A dose-finding approach based on shrunken predictive probability for combinations of two agents in phase I trials. Stat. Med. **32**, 4515–4525 (2013)

Hirakawa, A., Sato, H., Gosho, M.: Effect of design specifications in dose-finding trials for combination therapies in oncology. Pharm. Stat. **15**, 531–540 (2016)

Hirakawa, A., Sato, H.: Authors' reply. Stat. Med. **35**, 479–480 (2016)

Hirakawa, A., Wages, N.A., Sato, H., Matsui, S.: A comparative study of adaptive dose-finding designs for phase I oncology trials of combination therapies. Stat. Med. **34**, 3194–3213 (2015)

Hwang, J., Peddada, S.D.: Confidence interval estimation subject to order restrictions. Ann. Stat. **22**, 67–93 (1994)

Iasonos, A., Wilton, A.S., Riedel, E.R., Seshan, V.E., Spriggs, D.R.: A comprehensive comparison of the continual reassessment method to the standard 3+3 dose escalation scheme in phase 1 dose-finding studies. Clin. Trials **5**, 465–477 (2008)

Ivanova, A., Kim, S.H.: Dose finding for continuous and ordinal outcomes with a monotone objective function: a unified approach. Biometrics **65**, 307–315 (2009)

Ivanova, A., Wang, K.: A non-parametric approach to the design and analysis of two-dimensional dose-finding trials. Stat. Med. **23**, 1861–1870 (2004)

Jones, D.R., Moskaluk, C.A., Gillenwater, H.H., Petroni, G.R., Burks, S.G., Philips, J., Rehm, P.K., Olazagasti, J., Kozower, B.D., Bao, Y.: Phase I trial of induction histone deacetylase and proteasome inhibition followed by surgery in non-small-cell lung cancer. J. Thorac. Oncol. **7**, 1683–1690 (2012)

Kakurai, Y., Hirakawa, A., Hamada, C.: A dose-finding method based on multiple dosing in two-agent combination phase I trials. J. Biopharm. Stat. **25**, 1065–1076 (2015)

Kim, K.B., Alrwas, A.: Treatment of KIT-mutated metastatic mucosal melanoma. Chin. Clin. Oncol. **3**, 35 (2014)

Lee, S.M., Cheung, Y.K.: Model calibration in the continual reassessment method. Clin. Trials **6**, 227–238 (2009)

Mander, A.P., Sweeting, M.J.: A product of independent beta probabilities dose escalation design for dual-agent phase I trials. Stat. Med. **34**, 1261–1276 (2015)

Marusyk, A., Almendro, V., Polyak, K.: Intra-tumour heterogeneity: a looking glass for cancer? Nat. Rev. Cancer **12**, 323–334 (2012)

O'Quigley, J., Pepe, M., Fisher, L.: Continual reassessment method: a practical design for phase I clinical trials in cancer. Biometrics **46**, 33–48 (1990)

O'Quigley, J., Zohar, S.: Retrospective robustness of the continual reassessment method. J. Biopharm. Stat. **20**, 1013–1025 (2010)

Riviere, M.K., Yuan, Y., Dubois, F., Zohar, S.: A Bayesian dose-finding design for drug combination clinical trials based on the logistic model. Pharm. Stat. **13**, 247–257 (2014)

Sweeting, M.J., Mander, A.P.: Escalation strategies for combination therapy phase I trials. Pharm. Stat. **11**, 258–266 (2012)

Thall, P.F., Millikan, R.E., Mueller, P., Lee, S.J.: Dose-finding with two agents in phase I oncology trials. Biometrics **59**, 487–496 (2003)

Wages, N.A., Conaway, M.R.: Specifications of a continual reassessment method design for phase I trials of combined drugs. Pharm. Stat. **12**, 217–224 (2013)

Wages, N.A., Conaway, M.R., O'Quigley, J.: Continual reassessment method for partial ordering. Biometrics **67**, 1555–1563 (2011a)

Wages, N.A., Conaway, M.R., O'Quigley, J.: Dose-finding design for multi-drug combinations. Clin. Trials **8**, 380–389 (2011b)

Wages, N.A., Varhegyi, N.: POCRM: an R-package for phase I trials of combinations of agents. Comput. Methods Programs Biomed. **112**, 211–218 (2013)

Wang, K., Ivanova, A.: Two-dimensional dose finding in discrete dose space. Biometrics **61**, 217–222 (2005)

Yin, G., Yuan, Y.: A latent contingency table approach to dose finding for combinations of two agents. Biometrics **65**, 866–875 (2009a)

Yin, G., Yuan, Y.: Bayesian dose finding for drug combinations by copula regression. Appl. Stat. **58**, 211–224 (2009b)

Chapter 3
Dose Finding for Joint Assessment of Both Efficacy and Toxicity

Abstract Traditionally, phase I trials are designed to determine the MTD of a new agent based solely on toxicity, regardless of the efficacy. The determination of an optimal dose based on the joint assessment of toxicity and efficacy of the drug in phase I dose-finding trials may be reasonable in some cases. The various types of incorporation of toxicity and efficacy outcomes into dose-finding methods have been developed. Among them, in this chapter, we overview four methods: (i) the bivariate continual reassessment method, (ii) Bayesian method based on the efficacy–toxicity trade-off, (iii) Bayesian method for evaluating binary toxicity and continuous efficacy outcomes, and (iv) the method based on the Bayesian Model Averaging (BMA).

Keywords Bivariate · Correlation · Efficacy and toxicity · Joint assessment

3.1 Introduction

For cytotoxic agents, increased exposure to a drug augments tumor cell killing in preclinical models. This dose–response relationship in preclinical models is extrapolated to humans, as a consequence of which "the more the better" approach (i.e., the more toxic the treatment, the stronger effect we anticipate seeing) has become one of the most popular in oncology (Postel-Vinay et al. 2009; Sleijfer and Wiemer 2008). Thus, safety is first examined in a phase I trial, in which dose-finding methods are aimed at estimating the MTD of a new drug, fulfilling ethical constraints by minimizing the number of patients treated at too toxic levels. Then, efficacy of the MTD is typically examined in a subsequent phase II trial.

Nonetheless, some cancer therapies, such as cancer vaccines, are generally much safer than cytotoxic agents, and the dose that yields a sufficient biological activity is unlikely to confer significant toxicity. Hence, for these therapies, ethical concerns have been extended to the additional constraint that the proportion of patients who receive an ineffective dose can be minimized. In addition, due to statistical and resource insufficiency of the traditional two-phase approach (i.e., the safety and efficacy of a new agent is studied sequentially in phases I and II, respectively), various

© The Author(s), under exclusive licence to Springer Japan KK, part of Springer Nature 2018   41
A. Hirakawa et al., *Modern Dose-Finding Designs for Cancer Phase I Trials:*
Drug Combinations and Molecularly Targeted Agents, JSS Research Series
in Statistics, https://doi.org/10.1007/978-4-431-55573-5_3

dose-finding methods taking into account toxicity and efficacy simultaneously have been developed for clinical trials.

Gooley et al. (1994) were perhaps the first to consider two dose–outcome curves using a simulation as a design tool. They discussed the design and analysis of a proposed phase I/II clinical trial for a bone marrow transplant. That design sought a dose that balanced the risks of two immunological complications. Thall and Russell (1998) proposed a phase I/II design to find a dose that would satisfy both safety and efficacy requirements based on a trinary outcome. They used a proportional odds model (McCullagh 1989) to model the dose–outcome relationship. Thall and Cook (2004) developed a Bayesian phase I/II trial design based on trade-offs between efficacy and toxicity probabilities. They proposed to use the Gumbel model (Murtaugh and Fisher 1990) to capture the relation between the bivariate binary toxicity and efficacy outcomes. They employed the quadratic model for the dose–efficacy relationship to consider a nonmonotonic pattern.

As an extension of the CRM, Braun (2002) proposed the bivariate CRM that accounts for both toxicity and efficacy outcomes. Their work was motivated by research into allogeneic stem cell transplantation for older and advanced leukemia patients. Asakawa et al. (2014) devised a way to incorporate the BMA into the bivariate CRM to accommodate the misspecification of the true dose–toxicity and dose–efficacy relationships of the drug.

The above methods have been developed for binary toxicity and efficacy outcomes, but we often encounter a situation where the efficacy is measured as a continuous variable such as pharmacodynamic markers in practice. Bekele and Shen (2005) utilized bivariate probit models, in which a patient's toxicity and efficacy outcomes correlate with each other to develop the dose-finding method to explain binary toxicity and continuous efficacy outcomes. A continuous latent variable was introduced for the joint modeling of the continuous efficacy and the binary toxicity outcomes in a bivariate model, at each given dose level. Similarly, Hirakawa (2012) proposed a dose-finding method for analysis of correlating bivariate binary toxicity and continuous efficacy outcomes by means of the factorization models in single-agent and two-agent combination trials.

In this chapter, we overview the four methods: (i) the bivariate CRM (Brawn, 2002), (ii) Bayesian method based on the efficacy–toxicity trade-off (Thall and Cook 2004), (iii) Bayesian method for evaluating binary toxicity and continuous efficacy outcomes (Hirakawa 2012), and (iv) the CRM-based method derived from BMA (Asakawa et al. 2014).

Hereafter, we mainly introduce both the statistical model for capturing the dose–efficacy and dose–toxicity relationships along with the dose-finding algorithm for exploring the optimal dose because almost all the dose-finding methods have often been developed by improving or devising these components. The notations of each method are independently defined because the models and dose-finding algorithm of each method are greatly different.

3.2   The Bivariate Continual Reassessment Method

Braun (2002) attempted to find a regimen that is optimal, in the sense that acute graft-versus-host disease and disease progression rates are both kept near desired thresholds.

3.2.1   Modeling Toxicity and Efficacy Outcomes

For each subject i $(i = 1, \cdots, N)$, let Y_i and Z_i be the indicators of toxicity and progression (that is no efficacy). Y_i (or Z_i) $= 1$ indicates that toxicity (or progression) is observed, and Y_i (or Z_i) $= 0$ indicates otherwise.

The respective probabilities of toxicity and progression, $\pi_Y(d_l)$ and $\pi_Z(d_l)$, are associated with each dose d_l $(l = 1, \cdots, L)$ via the equations

$$\pi_Y(d_l) = \frac{\exp(-3 + \beta_1 d_l)}{1 + \exp(-3 + \beta_1 d_l)}, \tag{3.1}$$

$$\pi_Z(d_l) = \frac{\exp(3 - \beta_2 d_l)}{1 + \exp(3 - \beta_2 d_l)}. \tag{3.2}$$

Braun (2002) assumed that each pair (Y_i, Z_i) has a bivariate distribution;

$$f(y, z \mid d) = C\pi_Y^y (1 - \pi_Y)^{(1-y)} \pi_Z^z (1 - \pi_Z)^{(1-z)} \psi^{yz} (1 - \psi)^{(1-yz)} \tag{3.3}$$

where ψ denotes the association between Y and Z, and C is a normalizing constant. Thus, the parameter vector is given by $\theta = (\beta_1, \beta_2, \psi)$ in this dose-finding method.

After we observe the results for a cohort of n subjects, D_n, the likelihood is given by

$$\mathcal{L}(\theta \mid D_n) = \prod_{i=1}^{n} f(y_i, z_i). \tag{3.4}$$

Braun (2002) presumed a noninformative prior for θ, $p(\theta)$, specifically,

$$p(\theta) = 6\psi(1 - \psi)\exp\{-(\beta_1 + \beta_2)\}, \ \beta_1 > 0, \ \beta_2 > 0, \ 0 < \psi < 1 \tag{3.5}$$

which applies an exponential distribution with a mean of 1 to each regression parameter β_1, β_2, and a beta distribution with the mean 0.5 to association parameter ψ. Note that β_1, β_2, and ψ are assumed to be marginally independent.

The posteriors of θ are expressed as

$$p(\theta \mid D_n) \propto \mathcal{L}(\theta \mid D_n)p(\theta). \tag{3.6}$$

Braun (2002) estimated the posterior mean of θ by the integral approximation method proposed by Tierney and Kadane (1986).

3.2.2　The Dose-Finding Algorithm

Definition of the Optimal Dose:

Braun (2002) defined the optimal dose as the dose that minimized the Euclidean distance u_l of the posterior probabilities $(\hat{\pi}_Y(d_l), \hat{\pi}_Z(d_l))$ to the target rates of toxicity and progression (π_Y^*, π_Z^*) at the end of the study:

$$u_l = \sqrt{(\hat{\pi}_Y(d_l) - \pi_Y^*)^2 + (\hat{\pi}_Z(d_l) - \pi_Z^*)^2}. \tag{3.7}$$

Acceptable Dose Criteria:

To control the risk of treating subjects at a dose with either unacceptably high toxicity or unacceptably low efficacy, Braun (2002) placed a limit on the dose escalation/de-escalation based on the lower bound of a one-sided 95% confidence interval for the overall rate of toxicity LB_Y and for the overall rate of disease progression LB_Z. LB_Y and LB_Z are estimated from the total toxic events e_Y and total progression events e_Z among n subjects. The specific dose escalation/de-escalation rules will be described later.

Dose-Finding Algorithm:

In their dose-finding method, a first cohort with c subjects is treated at the starting dose that the investigator considers the optimal dose. After n subjects have been enrolled, using the posterior mean of θ, we calculate the posterior probabilities of toxicity and progression outcomes for each dose, $\hat{\pi}_Y(d_l)$ and $\hat{\pi}_Z(d_l)$. The dose allocated to the next cohort of patients is determined as follows:

1. If $LB_Y \leq \pi_Y^*$ and $LB_Z \leq \pi_Z^*$, the dose corresponding to the smallest value of u_l is selected, and a new cohort of c subjects enters on that dose.
2. If $LB_Y > \pi_Y^*$ and $LB_Z \leq \pi_Z^*$, then patients of the next cohort will be treated at the dose that minimized u_l only if that dose is lower than the current dose. Otherwise, the dose will be decreased to the next lowest dose from the current dose.
3. If $LB_Y \leq \pi_Y^*$ and $LB_Z > \pi_Z^*$, then patients of the next cohort will be treated at the dose that minimized u_l only if it is higher than the current dose. Otherwise, the dose will be escalated to the next highest dose.

This procedure is repeated until the maximum number of patients N have been enrolled, and then we determine the optimal dose. If both confidence intervals LB_Y and LB_Z lie above the target rates or their dose-finding method recommends increasing above dose d_L or decreasing below dose d_1, then the study will be terminated early.

3.2.3 Operating Characteristics

Braun (2002) compared the performance of the bivariate CRM with that of the designs proposed by Gooley et al. (1994) in simulation studies under three scenarios. Gooley et al. (1994) proposed three rule-based dose-finding designs, denoted as designs A–C, based on the number of patients without efficacy (rejection after a transplant) or with toxicity. The dose-finding algorithms of the three designs are quite similar. The major differences among the three designs are the criteria for increasing or decreasing the dose level. For further details, see the original paper. According to the simulation results published by Gooley et al. (1994), the operating characteristics of design A were deemed inferior to those of designs B and C. Therefore, we focused on designs B and C, and compared the operating characteristics among the bivariate CRM and designs B and C.

Braun (2002) assumed 18 dose levels and 60 patients in total. The first cohort of patients was allocated to dose level 14. The outcomes of each subject were simulated to be negatively associated with $\psi = 1/2$. Each simulation consisted of 1,000 trials.

In the two scenarios, which include more than two true optimal doses, the means of the recommended rates for the true optimal dose of the bivariate CRM, design B, and design C were 67.0%, 61.6%, and 77.1%, and the mean termination rates of the study on the bivariate CRM, design B, and design C were 23.9%, 24.7%, and 13.7%, respectively. In the scenarios in which no optimal dose exists, the bivariate CRM, design B, and design C revealed termination rates of the trial, 92.3%, 85.3%, and 76.7%, and average numbers of subjects per trial of the bivariate CRM, design B, and design C were 19.6, 25.6, and 27.9, respectively.

Judging by these simulation results, the average performance of the bivariate CRM was slightly higher than that of design B but lower than that of design C by approximately 10% of the recommended rates for a true optimal dose. On the other hand, the bivariate CRM terminated the study earlier than design B and design C when no optimal dose exists. Thus, the bivariate CRM can be considered a more conservative method than design C.

3.2.4 Software Implementation

A software package for implementing the bivariate CRM can be downloaded from https://biostatistics.mdanderson.org/softwaredownload/SingleSoftware.aspx?-Software_Id=15.

When applying the bivariate CRM, we input (i) monitoring outcomes (Toxicity/Efficacy/Toxicity and Efficacy), (ii) a definition of a true optimal dose (the target rates of toxicity; the target rates of efficacy; the closest dose to the target/the dose above the target/the dose below the target), (iii) the value of the intercept parameter in the toxicity–efficacy model [-3 in Eq. (3.1) and 3 in Eq. (3.2)], (iv) the number of dose levels, (v) initial dose level, (vi) maximum dose-level increment, (vii) the range of toxicity and efficacy probability (minimum and maximum probabilities of toxicity and efficacy), (viii) cohort size, and (ix) minimum and maximum sample sizes. Note that it is necessary to use the reciprocal of disease progression rates in Eq. (3.2) when we input (iii), the value of the intercept parameter, into the efficacy model (i.e., input the value of -3 instead of 3).

After we run simulations, the main program window can show the summary data for the different scenarios and design variants simulated.

3.3 Dose Finding Based on Efficacy–Toxicity Trade-Offs

Thall and Cook (2004) developed a Bayesian phase I/II trial design based on the efficacy–toxicity trade-offs that a physician would consider desirable. The models for bivariate binary and trinary outcomes are considered in this dose-finding method. Here, we introduce only the model for bivariate binary outcomes.

3.3.1 Modeling Toxicity and Efficacy Outcomes

Let Y_{Ei} and Y_{Ti} be the indicators of efficacy and toxicity for the ith patient ($i = 1, \cdots, N$). Y_{Ei} (or Y_{Ti}) $= 1$ indicates that efficacy (or toxicity) is observed, and Y_{Ei} (or Y_{Ti}) $= 0$ indicates otherwise. Given the actual L doses $d_1, \cdots, d_L$, standardized dose $d_l' = \log(d_l) - L^{-1} \sum_{m=1}^{L} d_m$, ($l = 1, \cdots, L$) is used for the models underlying the dose-finding method.

Thall and Cook (2004) formulated the marginal probability of toxicity $\pi_T(d_l')$ and efficacy $\pi_E(d_l')$ as follows:

$$\pi_T(d_l') = \frac{\exp(\alpha_T + \beta_T d_l')}{1 + \exp(\alpha_T + \beta_T d_l')}, \tag{3.8}$$

$$\pi_E(d_l') = \frac{\exp\left(\alpha_E + \beta_{E,1} d_l' + \beta_{E,2} d_l'^2\right)}{1 + \exp\left(\alpha_E + \beta_{E,1} d_l' + \beta_{E,2} d_l'^2\right)}. \tag{3.9}$$

The joint probability function for Y_{Ei} and Y_{Ti} is modeled by the Gumbel model:

$$\begin{aligned}
\pi_{a,b}(x_i, \theta) &= \Pr(Y_{Ei} = a, Y_{Ti} = b | x_i, \theta) \\
&= (\pi_E)^a (1 - \pi_E)^{1-a} (\pi_T)^b (1 - \pi_T)^{1-b} \\
&\quad + (-1)^{a+b} \pi_E (1 - \pi_E) \pi_T (1 - \pi_T) \left(\frac{e^\psi - 1}{e^\psi + 1}\right)
\end{aligned} \tag{3.10}$$

for $a, b \in \{0, 1\}$, where x_i and ψ denote the actual dose administered to patient i and the association parameter, respectively. Thus, the parameter vector is given by $\theta = \left(\alpha_T, \beta_T, \alpha_E, \beta_{E,1}, \beta_{E,2}, \psi\right)$ in this dose-finding method.

If we denote the data for the first n patients in the trial as D_n, then the likelihood is given by

$$\mathcal{L}_n \left(\theta \mid D_n \right) = \prod_{i=1}^{n} \prod_{a=0}^{1} \prod_{b=0}^{1} \left\{ \pi_{a,b} \left(x_i, \theta \right) \right\}^{I\{Y_i=(a,b)\}}. \tag{3.11}$$

Thall and Cook (2004) assumed that each component of θ has a normal distribution, i.e., $\alpha_T \sim N \left(\tilde{\mu}_{\alpha_T}, \tilde{\sigma}_{\alpha_T} \right), \beta_T \sim N \left(\tilde{\mu}_{\beta_T}, \tilde{\sigma}_{\beta_T} \right), \alpha_E \sim N \left(\tilde{\mu}_{\alpha_E}, \tilde{\sigma}_{\alpha_E} \right), \beta_{E,1} \sim N \left(\tilde{\mu}_{\beta_{E,1}}, \tilde{\sigma}_{\beta_{E,1}} \right), \beta_{E,2} \sim N \left(\tilde{\mu}_{\beta_{E,2}}, \tilde{\sigma}_{\beta_{E,2}} \right), \psi \sim N \left(\tilde{\mu}_{\psi}, \tilde{\sigma}_{\psi} \right)$, respectively. Suppose $\xi = \left(\tilde{\mu}_{\alpha_T}, \tilde{\sigma}_{\alpha_T}, \cdots, \tilde{\mu}_{\psi}, \tilde{\sigma}_{\psi} \right)$ denotes the vector of hyperparameters with all prior covariance sets equal to 0, and let $\phi \left(\theta \mid \xi \right)$ denote the normal prior of θ.

The posteriors of θ are given by

$$\phi(\theta \mid \xi, D_n) \propto \mathcal{L}_n \left(\theta \mid D_n \right) \phi(\theta \mid \xi). \tag{3.12}$$

By the method of Monahan and Genz (1997), Thall and Cook (2004) numerically integrated $\mathcal{L}_n \left(D_n \mid \theta \right) \phi(\theta \mid \xi)$ with respect to θ for computing the posteriors.

To establish the value of hyperparameters, for each dose d'_l, Thall and Cook (2004) considered the prior mean of $\pi_E \left(d'_l \right)$, denoted as $m_{E,l}(\xi)$ and $m_{T,l}(\xi)$, and the prior standard deviations of $\pi_E \left(d'_l \right)$ and $\pi_T \left(d'_l \right)$, denoted as $s_{E,l}(\xi)$ and $s_{T,l}(\xi)$. Additionally, Thall and Cook (2004) proposed to specify the values of the target means $m^*_{E,l}$ and $m^*_{T,l}$ based on the physician's opinion, and the values of the target standard deviations $s^*_{E,l}$ and $s^*_{T,l}$ in the range 0.29–0.50. Then, by the Nelder–Mead algorithm (Nelder and Mead 1965), we numerically solved for the value of ξ that best fits the target means and variances by minimizing the objective function

$$h(\xi) = \sum_{y=E,T} \sum_{1 \le l \le L} \left[\left\{ m_{y,l}(\xi) - m^*_{y,l} \right\}^2 + \left\{ s_{y,l}(\xi) - s^*_{y,l} \right\}^2 \right] + c \sum_{1 \le l \le k \le L} (\tilde{\sigma}_l - \tilde{\sigma}_k)^2. \tag{3.13}$$

The second term in $h(\xi)$ is included so that the solution will distribute the prior variance more evenly among the components of θ, with c being a small positive constant.

3.3.2 The Dose-Finding Algorithm

The Definition of the Optimal Dose:

Thall and Cook (2004) considered the situation where the dose-finding method based on the Euclidean distance from the point of interest to the most desirable point, $(\pi_E, \pi_T) = (1, 0)$ may not reflect clinical desirable outcomes in practice because this method puts equal weight on efficacy and toxicity. Instead of using the Euclidean distance, Thall and Cook (2004) developed a new indicator, which is designated as "desirability," to identify the optimal dose based on the efficacy–toxicity trade-offs that a physician would consider desirable.

At first, to calculate the desirability, we have to establish the target efficacy–toxicity trade-off contour, C, such that all the points on C are equally desirable.

The way to construct C is introduced in the next subsection. Once the trade-off contour C is established, for each given dose level, we obtain an intersection point $Z = \left(\pi_{Ez} \left(d_l' \right), \pi_{Tz} \left(d_l' \right) \right)$ of the trade-off contour and a straight line that cuts across the points of the posterior efficacy and toxicity probabilities $\left(\hat{\pi}_E \left(d_l' \right), \hat{\pi}_T \left(d_l' \right) \right)$ and the ideal efficacy and toxicity probability pair $(1, 0)$. Thus, the desirability value for $d_l', \delta \left(d_l' \right)$, is defined as follows:

$$\delta \left(d' \right) = \frac{\sqrt{\left(\pi_{Ez} \left(d_l' \right) - 1 \right)^2 + \left(\pi_{Tz} \left(d_l' \right) - 0 \right)^2}}{\sqrt{\left(\hat{\pi}_E \left(d_l' \right) - 1 \right)^2 + \left(\hat{\pi}_T \left(d_l' \right) - 0 \right)^2}} - 1 \qquad (3.14)$$

If $\left(\hat{\pi}_E \left(d_l' \right), \hat{\pi}_T \left(d_l' \right) \right)$ is on the trade-off contour, then the desirability value is 0. The larger positive desirability value indicates a more desirable dose level.

Acceptable Dose Criteria:

Thall and Cook (2004) defined the minimum efficacy and maximum toxicity criteria as follows:

$$\Pr \left\{ \pi_E \left(d', \theta \right) > \overline{\pi}_E | D_n \right\} > p_E, \qquad (3.15)$$

$$\Pr \left\{ \pi_T \left(d', \theta \right) < \underline{\pi}_T | D_n \right\} > p_T, \qquad (3.16)$$

where $\overline{\pi}_E$ and $\underline{\pi}_T$ are fixed lower and upper limits specified by the physician, and p_E and p_T are fixed probability cutoffs. The probability cutoffs p_E and p_T may be determined, from preliminary computer simulation results, to obtain a design with desirable operating characteristics. If d' satisfies both Eqs. (3.15) and (3.16), or if d' is the lowest untried dose above the starting dose and satisfies Eq. (3.16), then d' is an acceptable dose.

The Dose-Finding Algorithm:

We treat the first cohort at the starting dose specified by the physician. During the trial, after the most recent cohort's data have been incorporated into D_n, the desirability for each $d_l', \delta \left(d_l' \right)$, is calculated, and the dose—that maximizes $\delta \left(d_l' \right)$ among the doses with acceptable efficacy and toxicity—is to be administered to the next cohort of patients. This procedure is repeated until the maximum number of patients N is reached. At this point, there is at least one acceptable dose, then dose d' among acceptable doses maximizing $\delta \left(d_l' \right)$ is selected as the optimal dose. If there are no acceptable doses, then the trial is terminated early and no dose is selected.

3.3.3 Constructing a Trade-Off Contour

To construct C, three target values, $\left\{ \pi_1^*, \pi_2^*, \pi_3^* \right\}$, that the physician considers equally desirable, are elicited. First, we elicit a desirable trade-off target, $\pi_1^* = \left(\pi_{1,E}^*, \pi_{1,T}^* \right) =$

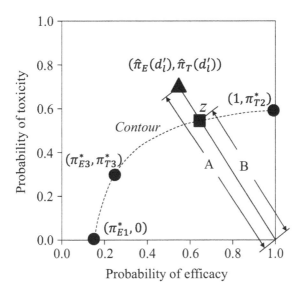

Fig. 3.1 The efficacy–toxicity trade-off contour is represented by the dotted curve. This contour is generated from the three equally desirable elicited target points $\left(\pi_{E1}^*,\ 0\right)$, $\left(1, \pi_{T2}^*\right)$, $\left(\pi_{E3}^*,\ \pi_{T3}^*\right)$, which are represented by filled circles. Z represented by a filled square is the intersection point of the trade-off contour and a straight line that cuts across the points of the posterior efficacy and toxicity probabilities $\left(\hat{\pi}_E\left(d_l'\right),\ \hat{\pi}_T\left(d_l'\right)\right)$ (represented by a filled triangle), and the ideal efficacy and toxicity probability pair $(1, 0)$. "A" is Euclidean distance from the point of $\left(\hat{\pi}_E\left(d_l'\right),\ \hat{\pi}_T\left(d_l'\right)\right)$ to optimal point $(1, 0)$, and "B" is Euclidean distance from the intersection point z to optimal point $(1, 0)$. The desirability value is defined as $B/A - 1$

$\left(\pi_{1,E}^*, 0\right)$, in the case where toxicity has probability 0. Next, we elicit π_2^* having the same desirability as π_1^* by asking the physician what the maximum value of π_T may be if in the bivariate binary outcome case $\pi_E = 1$. Given these two equally desirable extremes, we elicit a third pair, π_3^*, that is equally desirable but is intermediate between π_1^* and π_2^*. We plot each target as it is elicited and draw the target efficacy–toxicity trade-off contour, C, determined by $\left\{\pi_1^*, \pi_2^*, \pi_3^*\right\}$ (Fig. 3.1).

Thall and Cook (2004) used the convenient form $\pi_T = f\left(\pi_E\right) = a + b/\pi_E + c/\pi_E^2$ in their work, fitted to the three elicited target pairs subject to the constraint that f be nondecreasing for π_E such that $\left\{\pi_E, f\left(\pi_E\right)\right\} \in C$.

3.3.4 Operating Characteristics

Thall and Cook (2004) illustrated their dose-finding method's behavior in a simulation study under six scenarios. The number of dose levels was four, and the maximum sample size was set to 36. The starting dose was dose level 1, and the number of patients allocated to each dose level was set to 3. In each scenario, the efficacy and toxicity occurred independently (i.e., $\phi = 0$).

In addition, we set $\overline{\pi}_E = 0.20$, $\underline{\pi}_T = 0.40$, and $p_E = p_T = 0.10$. The means and standard deviations of the prior parameters were $(\tilde{\mu}_{\alpha_T}, \tilde{s}_{\alpha_T}) = (-0.619, 0.941)$, $(\tilde{\mu}_{\beta_T}, \tilde{s}_{\beta_T}) = (0.587, 1.659)$, $(\tilde{\mu}_{\alpha_E}, \tilde{s}_{\alpha_E}) = (-1.496, 1.113)$, $(\tilde{\mu}_{\beta_{E.1}}, \tilde{s}_{\beta_{E.1}}) = (1.180, 0.869)$, $(\tilde{\mu}_{\beta_{E.2}}, \tilde{s}_{\beta_{E.2}}) = (0.149, 1.192)$ and $(\tilde{\mu}_{\psi}, \tilde{s}_{\psi}) = (0, 1.00)$, respectively. To construct C, the three target values $(\pi_{E1}^*, 0)$, $(1, \pi_{T2}^*)$, $(\pi_{E3}^*, \pi_{T3}^*) = (0.15, 0)$, $(1, 0.60)$, $(0.25, 0.30)$ were selected.

As a result, in five scenarios, which include a true optimal dose, the mean of the recommended rates for the true optimal dose was 82.6%. In the scenario where no dose was acceptable, the trial was correctly stopped early with no dose selected 94.5% of the time. Thus, Thall and Cook (2004) demonstrated that their dose-finding method may be able to make a correct decision, namely, select the optimal dose or stop early when no doses are acceptable.

3.3.5   Software Implementation

Readers can use publicly released software EffTox (version 4.0.12), which can be downloaded from https://biostatistics.mdanderson.org/softwaredownload/-SingleSoftware.aspx?Software_Id=2.

To run EffTox, the essential inputs—(i) prior efficacy and toxicity probabilities for doses, (ii) effective sample size, (iii) equally desirable target efficacy–toxicity probability pairs, (iv) true efficacy and toxicity probabilities for each dose level, and (v) the conditional probability of efficacy given no toxicity outcome—are required but are not limited to these values.

Depending on prior efficacy and toxicity probabilities and effective sample size, the hyperparameters of the prior distribution with respect to the model parameters were automatically calculated. The prespecified efficacy–toxicity trade-off contour is also automatically constructed based on three determined efficacy and toxicity probability pairs that are considered by the physician to be equally desirable targets, that is, $\{\pi_1^*, \pi_2^*, \pi_3^*\}$.

3.4   A Bayesian Approach to Modeling Binary Toxicity and Continuous Efficacy Outcomes

Hirakawa (2012) developed a dose-finding method for evaluating continuous efficacy and binary toxicity outcomes in monotherapy and combination therapy. Here, we introduce only the model for monotherapy.

3.4.1 Modeling Toxicity and Efficacy Outcomes

Let Y_{Ti} and Y_{Ei}^* be a binary toxicity outcome and a raw continuous efficacy outcome for the ith of N patients. $Y_{Ti} = 1$ indicates that toxicity is observed, and $Y_{Ti} = 0$ indicates otherwise. A lower value of continuous efficacy outcome Y_{Ei}^* is regarded as superior to higher values.

Hirakawa (2012) assumed the probability of the toxicity outcome as follows:

$$\text{logit}\,(\pi_T\,(d_l)) = \log\left(\frac{\pi_T\,(d_l)}{1 - \pi_T\,(d_l)}\right) = \alpha_0 + \alpha_1 d_l, \tag{3.17}$$

where $\pi_T\,(d_l)$ is the probability of toxicity for dose $d_l, l = 1, \cdots, L$, and (α_0, α_1) are unknown parameters. Then, the distribution of Y_{Ti} matches the Bernoulli distribution, such that,

$$f\left(y_{Ti}|d_{l,i}\right) = \exp\left[y_{Ti}\psi_i - \log\{1 + \exp(\psi_i)\}\right], \tag{3.18}$$

where ψ_i equals $\text{logit}\,(\pi_{Ti})$, and $d_{l,i}$ denotes the actual dose for patient i.

For the continuous efficacy outcome, Hirakawa (2012) used the model previously described by O'Connell et al. (1993). A raw continuous efficacy outcome Y_{Ei}^* is transformed by $Y_{Ei} = h\left(Y_{Ei}^*\right)$, then the distribution of Y_{Ei} is normal with the mean μ_{Ei} and variance σ_i^2,

$$f\left(y_{Ei}|d_{l,i}\right) = \frac{1}{\sqrt{2\pi\sigma_i^2}}\exp\left\{-\frac{(y_{Ei} - \mu_{Ei})^2}{2\sigma_i^2}\right\}, \tag{3.19}$$

where

$$\mu_{Ei} = \beta_2 + \frac{\beta_1 - \beta_2}{1 + \left(d_{l,i}/\beta_3\right)^{\beta_4}}. \tag{3.20}$$

In this equation, $(\beta_1, \beta_2, \beta_3, \beta_4)$ are unknown parameters. Furthermore, as discussed by Harvey (1976), Hirakawa (2012) assumed variance σ_i^2 to be the multiplicative heteroscedasticity as follows:

$$\sigma_i^2 = \sigma^2 d_{l,i}^\lambda, \tag{3.21}$$

where σ^2 and λ are unknown parameters. The value of λ determines the degree of heteroscedasticity, particularly, homoscedasticity is held as the dose level increases when $\lambda = 0$.

Considering the correlation between binary toxicity and continuous efficacy outcomes, Hirakawa (2012) analyzed a model based on the factorization of the joint distribution of (Y_{Ti}, Y_{Ei}), which was previously introduced by Olkin and Tate (1961):

$$f\,(y_{Ti}, y_{Ei}) = f\,(y_{Ti})\,f\,(y_{Ei}|y_{Ti}). \tag{3.22}$$

The conditional distribution of y_{Ei} given y_{Ti} is normal,

$$f\left(y_{Ei}|y_{Ti}\right) = \frac{1}{\sqrt{2\pi\sigma_i^2}}\exp\left[-\frac{\{y_{Ei} - \mu_{Ei} - \tau\left(y_{Ti} - \pi_{Ti}\right)\}^2}{2\sigma_i^2}\right], \qquad (3.23)$$

where τ is the parameter for the regression of y_{Ei} on y_{Ti}. Large absolute values of τ indicate a strong correlation between the two outcomes. When $\tau = 0$, the two outcomes are independent given the dose level in the model. In this dose-finding method, parameter vector $\theta = \left\{\alpha_0, \alpha_1, \beta_1, \beta_2, \beta_3, \beta_4, \tau, \sigma^2, \lambda\right\}$

Given the current data D_n, the log-likelihood function is given by

$$\mathcal{L}(\theta|D_n) = \log\prod_{i=1}^{n} f\left(y_{bi}, y_{ci}|d_{l,i}\right) = \log\prod_{i=1}^{n} f\left(y_{ci}|y_{bi}, d_{l,i}\right) f\left(y_{bi}|d_{l,i}\right). \quad (3.24)$$

Hirakawa (2012) employed a Bayesian procedure to update the estimates of parameter vectors θ. In their work, the prior joint distributions for the parameter vectors of θ, $f(\theta)$, are an independent uniform distribution for each parameter.

In accordance with the Bayes theorem, the joint posterior distribution is

$$f(\theta|D_n) \propto f(\theta)\mathcal{L}(\theta|D_n). \qquad (3.25)$$

Hirakawa (2012) estimated the posterior means of θ by the random-walk Metropolis algorithm to generate a sequence of draws from the joint posterior distribution of parameters using the PROC MCMC in the SAS software, version 9.2 (SAS Institute Inc., Cary, NC, USA).

3.4.2 The Dose-Finding Algorithm

The Definition of the Optimal Dose:

Hirakawa (2012) defined the optimal dose as a dose level that has the minimum weighted Mahalanobis distance between the point of efficacy and toxicity outcomes and the optimal point $(y_{\min}, 0)$ among the dose levels whose efficacy and toxicity are acceptable. Specifically, to determine the optimal dose, Hirakawa (2012) used the posterior mean of the weighted Mahalanobis distance given by averaging the posterior samples. The kth posterior samples of the weighted Mahalanobis distance $(k = 1, \cdots, K)$ of the outcome $\left(\mu_E(d_l)^{(k)}, \pi_T(d_l)^{(k)}\right)$ to the optimal point $(y_{\min}, 0)$ are given by

$$m_l^{(k)} = \sqrt{\frac{c_1^2 A^2 + c_2^2 B^2 - 2\rho(d_l)^{(k)} c_1 c_2 AB}{1 - \{\rho(d_l)^{(k)}\}^2}}, \qquad (3.26)$$

where

$$A = \frac{y_{\min} - \mu_E \, (d_l)^{(k)}}{\sqrt{\tau^{2(k)} \rho \, (d_l)^{(k)} \left\{ 1 - \rho \, (d_l)^{(k)} \right\} + \sigma^{2(k)} d_l^{\lambda} \, (k)}}, \tag{3.27}$$

$$B = \frac{0 - \pi_T \, (d_l)^{(k)}}{\sqrt{p \, (d_l)^{(k)} \left\{ 1 - p \, (d_l)^{(k)} \right\}}}, \tag{3.28}$$

and $\rho \, (d_l)$ is the correlation between efficacy and toxicity, c_1 and c_2 are the pre-specified weight parameters for adjusting the trade-off between efficacy and toxicity, respectively. The posterior mean of the weighted Mahalanobis distance is calculated based on the posterior samples, that is,

$$\bar{m}_l = \frac{1}{K} \sum_{k=1}^{K} m_l^{(k)}. \tag{3.29}$$

When employing the Markov chain Monte Carlo method in the simulation studies, Hirakawa (2012) used a burn-in of 5,000 iterations with a chain of length 5,000, retaining every fifth sample. Therefore, the value of K is set to 1,000 throughout.

Acceptable Dose Criteria:

Hirakawa (2012) defined the acceptable dose levels as $T \, (d_l) = \{d_l | I \, [\mu_E \, (d_l) < \mu_0$ and $\pi_T \, (d_l) < \pi_0] = 1\}$, where $I \, [\cdot]$ is an indicator function, $\mu_E \, (d_l)$ and $\pi_T \, (d_l)$ are the posterior mean of the continuous efficacy and the posterior probability of a toxicity outcome for dose level $d_l \, (l = 1, \cdots, L)$, respectively. μ_0 and π_0 are critical values for the posterior estimates of $\mu_E \, (d_l)$ and $\pi_T \, (d_l)$, respectively.

The Dose-Finding Algorithm:

In this algorithm, c patients are allocated to a single dose level at a time, starting from the lowest dose level. If $T \, (d_l) \neq 0$, then the dose with the minimum value of $\bar{m}_l$ among $T \, (d_l)$ is allocated to the next patient until reaching the maximum number of patients N. At the end of the trial, we choose a dose level that has the minimum weighted Mahalanobis distance among $T \, (d_l)$ as an optimal dose. The trial is stopped early when $T \, (d_l) = 0$ for all dose levels and/or any of the following criteria is met:

$$\Pr \left\{ \hat{\pi}_T \, (d_1) > \pi_0 | Data \right\} > \delta_1, \tag{3.30}$$
$$\Pr \left\{ \hat{\mu}_E \, (d_L) > \mu_0 | Data \right\} > \delta_2, \tag{3.31}$$

where δ_1 and δ_2 are the prespecified threshold probabilities.

3.4.3 Operating Characteristics

Hirakawa (2012) compared the operating characteristics of the proposed method with those of the method published by Bekele and Shen (2005), through simulation studies under six scenarios. In this study, four dose levels were considered, and the maximum sample size N was set to 36. The starting dose was the lowest dose, and the number of patients allocated to the single dose c was set to 3. Hirakawa (2012) introduced a correlation between toxicity and efficacy into the simulations via a copula function. Here, we introduce the case of correlation coefficient $r = 0.2$, each simulation consisted of 1,000 trials.

The toxicity probability that is clinically allowed, π_0, was set to 0.3. The efficacy threshold that is clinically allowed, μ_0, was set to 1.1. In addition, the weight parameters c_1 and c_2 were both set to 1.0, and the probabilities δ_1 and δ_2 were both set to 0.7. Hirakawa (2012) used $\alpha_0 \sim Uniform\,(-10, 0)$, $\alpha_1 \sim Uniform\,(0, 5)$, $\beta_1 \sim Uniform\,(0, 10)$, $\beta_2 \sim Uniform\,(-10, 0)$, $\beta_3 \sim Uniform\,(0, 10)$, $\beta_4 \sim Uniform\,(0, 10)$, $\tau \sim Uniform\,(-10, 10)$, $\sigma^2 \sim Uniform\,(0, 10)$, and $\lambda \sim Uniform\,(-10, 10)$ for all the scenarios.

Under the four scenarios that include a true optimal dose, the mean of the recommended rates for the true optimal dose of Hirakawa's method and of Bekele and Shen's method were 85.3% and 82.0%, respectively. Under scenarios in which all four doses were unacceptable or had no efficacy, both methods did not select any of the four doses in more than 90% of the cases, but the average number of patients in the Hirakawa's method was 6.8, which was approximately a half of that of Bekele and Shen's method (13.9 patients).

3.5   The BMA Bivariate CRM

Asakawa et al. (2014) proposed to incorporate BMA into the bivariate CRM to mitigate the risk of the misspecification of the true dose–efficacy and dose–toxicity relationships of a drug.

3.5.1   Modeling Toxicity and Efficacy Outcomes

Suppose Y_{Ei} and Y_{Ti} are binary efficacy and toxicity outcomes for patient i ($i = 1, \cdots, N$). Y_{Ei} (or Y_{Ti}) $= 1$ indicates that efficacy (or toxicity) is observed, and Y_{Ei} (or Y_{Ti}) $= 0$ indicates otherwise.

Asakawa et al. (2014) presumed a power model for dose–efficacy and dose–toxicity relationships, which consist of the skeletons for efficacy and toxicity probability and unknown model parameters. To address misspecification of the true dose–efficacy and/or toxicity relationships, Asakawa et al. (2014) proposed to apply BMA, which estimates the posterior probability for toxicity and efficacy by averaging posterior probabilities. Thus, K working models, denoted as $WM_k\,(\pi_{Ek}\,(d_l)\,, \pi_{Tk}\,(d_l))$, ($k = 1, \cdots, K$), are prespecified for dose d_l ($l = 1, \cdots, L$). Working model WM_k is given by

$$\pi_{Ek}\left(d_l\right) = p_{Ekl}^{\exp\left(\beta_{Ek}\right)}, \tag{3.32}$$

$$\pi_{Tk}\left(d_l\right) = p_{Tkl}^{\exp\left(\beta_{Tk}\right)}, \tag{3.33}$$

where p_{Ekl} and p_{Tkl} are the kth skeletons for efficacy and toxicity probabilities at dose d_l, and β_{Ek} and β_{Tk} are unknown model parameters for the kth working model, respectively.

Suppose that n_l patients have been treated at dose d_l and z_{El} (or z_{Tl}) defined as the number of patients whose response is $Y_E = 1$ (or $Y_T = 1$) at dose d_l, respectively. In addition, z_l is defined as the number of patients whose response is $Y_E = 1$ and $Y_T = 1$ at dose d_l. For the observed data D, the likelihood function for WM_k is expressed as

$$\mathcal{L}(\beta_{Ek}, \beta_{Tk}, \psi_k, WM_k | D) \propto \prod_{l=1}^{L} \pi_{Ekl}^{z_{El}} \left(1 - \pi_{Ekl}\right)^{(n_l - z_{El})} \pi_{Tkl}^{z_{Tl}}$$

$$\left(1 - \pi_{Tkl}\right)^{(n_l - z_{Tl})} \psi_k^{z_l} \left(1 - \psi_k\right)^{(n_l - z_l)}, \tag{3.34}$$

where ψ_k is the association parameter.

The estimates of the parameter are updated by means of the Bayesian theorem. Asakawa et al. (2014) assumed the normal prior distribution $N\left(0, 4^2\right)$ for gradient parameters β_{Ek} and β_{Tk} and presumed beta distribution $Beta\left(2, 2\right)$ for association parameter ψ_k to have a prior mean value of 0.5 with sufficiently vague information.

Given the prior distribution, the joint posterior distribution is expressed as

$$f\left(\beta_{Ek}, \beta_{Tk}, \psi_k | D\right) \propto \mathcal{L}(\beta_{Ek}, \beta_{Tk}, \psi_k, WM_k | D) f\left(\beta_{Ek}\right) f\left(\beta_{Tk}\right) f\left(\psi_k\right). \tag{3.35}$$

Asakawa et al. (2014) estimated the posterior distribution of model parameters using a random-walk Metropolis algorithm to generate the sample for generating recursive draws from a particular Markov chain, whose stationary distribution is the same as the posterior joint distribution of parameters using PROC MCMC in SAS, version 9.2 (SAS Institute Inc., Cary, NC).

3.5.2 BMA Estimates

Let $\Pr\left(WM_k\right)$ be the prior probability that represents the prior relative certainty (or importance) for the kth working model with the restriction $\sum_k \Pr\left(WM_k\right) = 1$. In their work, each working model has equal prior probability. These probabilities for each working model are adaptively updated as posterior probabilities. The posterior model probability (PMP) is given by

$$\text{PMP}\,(WM_k) = \text{Pr}(WM_k|D) = \frac{\mathcal{L}(\beta_{Ek}, \beta_{Tk}, \psi_k, WM_k|D)\text{Pr}(WM_k)}{\sum_{m=1}^{K} \mathcal{L}(\beta_{Em}, \beta_{Tm}, \psi_m, WM_m|D)\text{Pr}(WM_m)}. \tag{3.36}$$

With PMP(WM_k) as a weight for the kth working model, the BMA estimates for efficacy and toxicity probabilities at the lth dose level are obtained simply as a weighted average of the posterior means of the efficacy and toxicity probability, $\hat{\pi}_{Ek}(d_l)$ and $\hat{\pi}_{Tk}(d_l)$, across K working models:

$$\bar{\pi}_E(d_l) = \sum_{k=1}^{K} \hat{\pi}_{Ek}(d_l)\,\text{PMP}\,(WM_k), \tag{3.37}$$

$$\bar{\pi}_T(d_l) = \sum_{k=1}^{K} \hat{\pi}_{Tk}(d_l)\,\text{PMP}\,(WM_k). \tag{3.38}$$

3.5.3   The Dose-Finding Algorithm

The Definition of the Optimal Dose:

Asakawa et al. (2014) defined an optimal dose as a dose level that minimizes the weighted Euclidean distance from the target efficacy and toxicity probabilities, (ϕ_E, ϕ_T), via BMA estimates of efficacy and toxicity probabilities, such that

$$ED_l = \sqrt{w(\phi_E - \bar{\pi}_{El})^2 + (1 - w)(\phi_T - \bar{\pi}_{Tl})^2}. \tag{3.39}$$

Asakawa et al. (2014) assumed $\phi_E = 1$ and $\phi_T = 0$ and $w = 0.5$, respectively.

Acceptable Dose Criteria:

To ensure at least minimal efficacy and maximal allowable toxicity with high probability, Asakawa et al. (2014) defined the minimum requirement criteria as follows:

$$\sum_{k=1}^{K} \text{Pr}(\hat{\pi}_{Ekl} \geq c_E)\text{PMP}(WM_k) \geq 0.9, \tag{3.40}$$

$$\sum_{k=1}^{K} \text{Pr}(\hat{\pi}_{Tkl} \leq c_T)\text{PMP}(WM_k) \geq 0.9, \tag{3.41}$$

where c_E and c_T are the critical values. Asakawa et al. (2014) set c_E and c_T to 0.2 and 0.3, respectively.

The Dose-Finding Algorithm:

In this dose-finding method, patients are allocated to a specific dose level in a cohort that consists of three patients. Among dose levels satisfying the above criteria, the dose level that minimizes ED_l is assigned to the next cohort of patients. It should be noted that the skipping a dose level during the escalation or de-escalation is not allowed. The trial is terminated when no dose levels satisfy these criteria. When the planned maximum number of patients is reached, then the optimal dose is determined by the BMA estimates of efficacy and toxicity probability based on all the accumulated outcomes.

3.5.4 Operating Characteristics

Asakawa et al. (2014) compared the operating characteristics of the proposed method with those of the ordinal bivariate CRM by means of each working model under eight scenarios. Asakawa et al. (2014) assumed five dose levels, and the maximum number of patients was set to 45. The patients were allocated to a specific dose level in a cohort that consists of three patients. The true correlation coefficient between these outcomes was assumed to be 0.5 on the scale of bivariate normal outcomes. Next, 1,000 simulations were conducted for each scenario. c_E and c_T were set to 0.2 and 0.3, $\phi_E = 1$ and $\phi_T = 0$, and $w = 0.5$, respectively. The prior distributions of parameters β_{Ek} and β_{Tk} were $N\left(0, 4^2\right)$, and the beta distribution $Beta\ (2, 2)$ was assumed to be the prior distribution of association parameter ψ_k. In that simulation study, four sets of working models for efficacy and toxicity probabilities were considered.

In six scenarios, which include a true optimal dose, the means of the recommended rates for the true optimal dose of the proposed and bivariate CRM involving the best-fitting working model were 61.9% and 75.3%, respectively. The probability of correct optimal-dose selection with the proposed method was the second best among the candidate designs in most of the cases. The differences in the correct optimal dose selection probabilities between the best-fitting working model and the proposed method were 7.4–39.1%. Under the scenarios where no dose was acceptable, the proposed method was correctly stopped early with no dose selected more than 90% of the time.

According to the simulations, if true dose–efficacy and dose–toxicity relationships for an investigational drug can be speculated based on prior information, then the ordinal bivariate CRM involving the working model corresponding to true dose–efficacy/toxicity relationships should be used. Nonetheless, in the cases without prior information about dose–efficacy and dose–toxicity relationships, the proposed method may be a useful alternative.

3.5.5 Software Implementation

Readers can use the BMA-based bivariate CRM method in SAS version 9.2. The SAS code to run this method (BMA-bCRM.sas) and estimate model parameters

(MCMC.sas) are available on the website http://www.rs.kagu.tus.ac.jp/hamada/lab. html.

To execute BMA-bCRM.sas, it is necessary to use MCMC.sas in BMA-bCRM.sas. Given the skeletons for efficacy probability and toxicity probability of each working model, a prior probability of each working model, and the minimum efficacy or maximum allowable toxicity criteria, BMA-bCRM.sas applies the BMA-based bivariate CRM to the input SAS dataset and outputs the dose level assigned to the next cohort of patients. The input SAS dataset must contain each patient's data on outcomes: an indicator of the toxicity outcome, indicator of the efficacy outcome, and the dose level used for the treatment.

References

Asakawa, T., Hirakawa, A., Hamada, C.: Bayesian model averaging continual reassessment method for bivariate binary efficacy and toxicity outcomes in phase I oncology trials. J. Biopharm. Stat. **24**, 310–325 (2014)

Bekele, B.N., Shen, Y.: A Bayesian approach to jointly modeling toxicity and biomarker expression in a phase I/II dose-finding trial. Biometrics **61**, 344–354 (2005)

Braun, T.M.: The bivariate continual reassessment method: extending the CRM to phase I trials of two competing outcomes. Control. Clin. Trials **23**, 240–256 (2002)

Gooley, T.A., Martin, P.J., Fisher, L.D., Pettinger, M.: Simulation as a design tool for phase I/II clinical trials: an example from bone marrow transplantation. Control. Clin. Trials **15**, 450–462 (1994)

Harvey, A.C.: Estimating regression models with multiplicative heteroscedasticity. Econometrica **44**, 461–465 (1976)

Hirakawa, A.: An adaptive dose-finding approach for correlated bivariate binary and continuous outcomes in phase I oncology trials. Stat. Med. **31**, 516–532 (2012)

McCullagh, P.: Models for discrete multivariate responses. Bull. Int. Stat. Inst. **53**, 407–418 (1989)

Monahan, J., Genz, A.: Spherical-radial integration rules for Bayesian computation. J. Am. Stat. Assoc. **92**, 664–674 (1997)

Murtaugh, P.A., Fisher, L.D.: Bivariate binary models of efficacy and toxicity in dose-ranging trials. Commun. Stat. Theory Methods **19**, 2003–2020 (1990)

Nelder, J.A., Mead, R.: A simplex method for function minimization. Comput. J. **7**, 308–313 (1965)

O'Connell, M.A., Belanger, B.A., Haaland, P.D.: Calibration and assay development using the four parameter logistic model. Chemom. Intell. Lab. Syst. **20**, 97–114 (1993)

Olkin, I., Tate, R.F.: Multivariate correlation models with mixed discrete and continuous variables. Ann. Math. Stat. **32**, 448–465 (1961)

Postel-Vinay, S., Arkenau, H.T., Olmos, D., Ang, J., Barriuso, J., Ashley, S., Banerji, U., De-Bono, J., Judson, I., Kaye, S.: Clinical benefit in Phase-I trials of novel molecularly targeted agents: does dose matter? Br. J. Cancer **100**, 1373–1378 (2009)

Sleijfer, S., Wiemer, E.: Dose selection in phase I studies: why we should always go for the top. J. Clin. Oncol. **26**, 1576–1578 (2008)

Thall, P.F., Cook, J.D.: Dose-finding based on efficacy-toxicity trade-offs. Biometrics **60**, 684–693 (2004)

Thall, P.F., Russell, K.E.: A strategy for dose-finding and safety monitoring based on efficacy and adverse outcomes in phase I/II clinical trials. Biometrics **54**, 251–264 (1998)

Tierney, L., Kadane, J.B.: Accurate approximations for posterior moments and marginal densities. J. Am. Stat. Assoc. **81**, 82–86 (1986)

Chapter 4
Dose Finding for Molecularly Targeted Agents (MTAs)

Abstract In the last 20 years, breakthroughs in the understanding of cancer cell biology resulted in the development of MTAs that are targeted to the unique genetics of each tumor and each patient. MTAs modulate specific aberrant pathways in cancer cells while sparing normal tissues, so that some MTAs do not necessarily need to be administered at their MTD to have maximal efficacy. Therefore, dose-finding methods that take into account the bivariate-correlating outcomes of both efficacy and toxicity are required for the clinical development of MTAs. In addition, the dose–efficacy model for MTAs is necessary to capture the specific relation between efficacy and the dose level. The efficacy may increase initially with the dose level but then reaches a plateau; however, this situation may not always be the case. Several powerful methods taking into account such a dose–efficacy relationship inherent in MTAs were devised recently. In this chapter, we overview the existing dose-finding methods intended to determine the optimal dose in singe-agent trials of MTAs.

Keywords Bivariate efficacy and toxicity · MTA · Optimal dose · Plateau

4.1 Introduction

MTAs modulate specific aberrant pathways in cancer cells while sparing normal tissues, and therefore most MTAs are expected to be more selective and less toxic than conventional cytotoxic drugs. Thus, the maximum therapeutic effect may be achieved at doses that are well below the MTD. This supposition comes from the results on clinical responses at different dose levels in clinical trials evaluating MTAs (Le Tourneau et al. 2015). In addition, the toxic effects of MTAs may manifest themselves through different mechanisms of action relative to the therapeutic effect, in which case, the toxic effects may not be predictive of the therapeutic effect (Fox et al. 2002). Therefore, dose-finding methods that evaluate efficacy and toxicity outcomes simultaneously are required for the clinical development of MTAs. In addition, the dose–efficacy model for MTAs should be able to capture the specific relation between efficacy and the dose level. In the dose–efficacy relationships of MTAs in most cases, the efficacy may increase initially with the dose level but then reaches a plateau;

© The Author(s), under exclusive licence to Springer Japan KK, part of Springer Nature 2018   59
A. Hirakawa et al., *Modern Dose-Finding Designs for Cancer Phase I Trials:*
Drug Combinations and Molecularly Targeted Agents, JSS Research Series
in Statistics, https://doi.org/10.1007/978-4-431-55573-5_4

however, this situation may not always be the case. Several dose-finding methods that take into account toxicity and efficacy simultaneously for determining the optimal dose in singe-agent trials were introduced in the previous chapter. Nevertheless, the efficacy model in these methods does not necessarily consider the dose–efficacy relationship inherent in MTAs.

To accommodate the dose–efficacy relationship of MTAs, Cai et al. (2014) proposed a logistic model with quadratic terms to capture the dose–efficacy relationship in the trials of combinations of biological agents. They regarded the shape of the dose–toxicity surface as initially monotonic with the dose escalation but changing to flat once it passes the threshold, and therefore, they selected a logistic model that reflects the fact that the dose–toxicity surface of combinations of biological agents may plateau. Riviere et al. (2015) incorporated a plateau parameter into a proportional hazards model for time to efficacy in a trial of a combination of a cytotoxic agent and an MTA. This approach also implies that after a certain dose level, the efficacy curve will plateau, even if toxicity is increasing. Wages and Tait (2015) proposed a power model for the binary efficacy outcome taking into account the notion that efficacy may decrease or reach a plateau after a certain dose level in a dose-finding trial of a single MTA. Sato et al. (2016) proposed a change point logistic model where the parameters change in the vicinity of the change point of the dose level. The change point is defined as the dose level at which the dose–efficacy pattern changes. Consequently, their method can capture various dose–efficacy patterns with an increase in the dose level. Riviere et al. (2016) selected the weighted likelihood approach to accommodate the possibility that efficacy has a late onset in the sense that efficacy takes a relatively long time to be assessed compared to toxicity (with respect to the accrual rate), such that when the next new patient arrives, patients who have enrolled into the trial have not completed their efficacy assessment yet. Those authors assumed that toxicity monotonically increases with the dose and modeled it via a logistic model.

In this chapter, we focus on three dose-finding methods, that is, those developed by Wages and Tait (2015), Sato et al. (2016), and Riviere et al. (2016). As described in the previous chapter, we first introduce the statistical models for capturing the dose–efficacy and dose–toxicity relationships as well as the dose-finding algorithm for analyzing the optimal dose. We also discuss the operating characteristics of each method. The symbols are independently defined by the dose-finding methods we introduce here because the models and dose-finding algorithm of each method are quite different.

4.2 The Model-Selecting Dose-Finding Method

Wages and Tait (2015) made use of some class of working models corresponding to unimodal or plateau dose–efficacy relationships for MTAs and continuously selected the model based on the posterior model probability through the trial.

4.2.1 Modeling Toxicity and Efficacy Outcomes

Let Y_i and Z_i denote binary toxicity and efficacy outcomes for the ith entering patient($i = 1, \ldots, N$), respectively. Y_i (or Z_i) = 1 indicates that toxicity (or efficacy) is observed, and Y_i (or Z_i) = 0 indicates otherwise. The dose for the ith entering patient, X_i, can be thought of as random, taking values $x_i \in \{d_1, \ldots, d_L\}$.

Wages and Tait (2015) formulated the toxicity probability as

$$\pi_T (d_l) = q_l^{\exp(\beta)}, \tag{4.1}$$

where q_l are skeletons representing discrete dose levels d_l. Wages and Tait (2015) assumed that toxicity monotonically increases with the dose; therefore, $0 < q_1 < \cdots < q_L < 1$. On the other hand, some class of working models for the efficacy probability is used to allow for more flexibility in modeling the dose–efficacy relationship. In this method, $K = 2 \times L - 1$ working models are prespecified; there are L unimodal skeletons and $L - 1$ plateau skeletons, which correspond to the dose–efficacy relationships where efficacy is increasing at low dose levels and either decreasing or plateauing at higher dose levels. For a particular skeleton, $k, k = 1, \ldots, K$, the true efficacy probability at d_l is modeled by

$$\pi_{Ek} (d_l) = p_{kl}^{\exp(\theta_k)}, \tag{4.2}$$

where p_{kl} is the skeleton of model k.

Wages and Tait (2015) estimated parameters β and θ_k based on the Bayesian framework. For the current data on n patients, D_n, to estimate parameters β and θ, the likelihood is given by

$$\mathcal{L} (\beta|D_n) = \prod_{i=1}^{n} \{\pi_T\}^{y_i} \{1 - \pi_T\}^{(1-y_i)} \text{ and} \tag{4.3}$$

$$\mathcal{L}_k (\theta_k|D_n) = \prod_{i=1}^{n} \{\pi_{Ek}\}^{z_i} \{1 - \pi_{Ek}\}^{(1-z_i)}, \text{ respectively.} \tag{4.4}$$

Wages and Tait (2015) utilized normal priors with mean 0 and variance 1.34 for β and θ_k as well as $g (\beta)$ and $h (\theta_k)$, respectively.

For $\mathcal{L} (\beta|D_n)$ and $\mathcal{L}_k (\theta_k|D_n)$, the posterior distributions of β and θ_k are given by

$$g (\beta|D_n) \propto g (\beta) \mathcal{L} (\beta|D_n) \text{ and} \tag{4.5}$$

$$h (\theta_k|D_n) \propto h (\theta_k) \mathcal{L}_k (\theta_k|D_n), \text{ respectively.} \tag{4.6}$$

Wages and Tait (2015) proposed to select the model based on the posterior model probability. Suppose $\Pr (Model_k)$ is a prior model probability for each possible skeleton. Based on the set D_n and the likelihood, posterior model probabilities

PMP $(Model_k)$ are as follows:

$$\text{PMP}\,(Model_k) = \text{Pr}\,(Model_k|D_n) = \frac{\text{Pr}\,(Model_k) \int \mathcal{L}_k\,(\theta_k|D_n)\,h\,(\theta_k)\,d\theta_k}{\sum_{m=1}^{K} \text{Pr}\,(Model_m) \int \mathcal{L}_m\,(\theta_m|D_n)\,h\,(\theta_m)\,d\theta_m}.$$

(4.7)

Each time a new patient is to be enrolled, Wages and Tait (2015) chose a single skeleton, k^*, with the largest posterior probability such that

$$k^* = \text{arg max}_k \text{PMP}\,(Model_k).$$

(4.8)

4.2.2 The Dose-Finding Algorithm

The Definition of the Optimal Dose:

Wages and Tait (2015) regarded an optimal dose as a dose level that has the maximum efficacy probability among the dose levels whose toxicity is acceptable.

Acceptable Dose Criteria:

Wages and Tait (2015) defined the acceptable set as follows:

$$T\,(d_l) = \left\{ d_l : \hat{\pi}_T\,(d_l) \le \phi_T \right\}$$

(4.9)

where $\pi_T\,(d_l)$ is the toxicity probability estimates for each dose, and ϕ_T is the critical value. It should be noted that Wages and Tait (2015) substituted the toxicity skeleton q_l for $\pi_T\,(d_l)$ to calculate $T\,(d_l)$ at the beginning of the trial.

The Dose-Finding Algorithm:

To accurately assign patients to the most efficacious dose with acceptable toxicity, early in the trial, Wages and Tait (2015) introduced an adaptive randomization phase. In this phase, the next cohort of patients is randomized to dose d_l with probability R_l, which is calculated from the estimated efficacy probabilities, $\hat{\pi}_E\,(d_l)$, for doses in $T\,(d_l)$, that is,

$$R_l = \frac{\hat{\pi}_E\,(d_l)}{\sum_{d_l \in T(d_l)} \hat{\pi}_E\,(d_l)}.$$

(4.10)

It should be noted that the first patient or cohort of patients is allocated to dose $x_1 = d_l$ with probability R_l based on the efficacy skeleton p_{kl}^* instead of $\hat{\pi}_E\,(d_l)$. This adaptive randomization phase is continued until a subset of n_R patients has been enrolled to allow information on untried doses to accumulate.

After the adaptive randomization phase, Wages and Tait (2015) initiated the maximization phase. The next cohort of patients is assigned to the dose level with the highest estimated efficacy probabilities, $\hat{\pi}_E\,(d_l)$ among the doses contained in $T\,(d_l)$. If we continue this way, then the optimal dose is the recommended dose after the inclusion of the maximum sample size of N patients.

In their dose-finding method, there are two stopping rules. Let $\pi_T^-(d_1)$ and ϕ_T be a lower bound of the 95% confidence interval for the probability of toxicity at d_1 and the maximum acceptable toxicity rate, respectively. In terms of safety, at any point in the trial, if $\pi_T^-(d_1) > \phi_T$, then we stop the trial for safety, and no treatment is identified as the optimal dose. In addition to the safety stopping rule, Wages and Tait (2015) set a futility stopping rule in the maximization phase. Suppose $\pi_E^+(x_n)$ and ϕ_E are an upper bound of the 95% confidence interval for the probability of efficacy at the current dose x_n and the futility threshold, respectively. If $\pi_E^+(x_n) < \phi_E$, then we stop the trial for futility, and no treatment is identified as the optimal dose.

4.2.3 Operating Characteristics

Wages and Tait (2015) compared the performance of the proposed method with that of the Hoering et al. method (2013) for identifying the optimal dose in simulations under 12 scenarios. The number of dose levels was six. The maximum sample size was set to 64, and the size of the adaptive randomization phase was set equal to one quarter of the total sample size. The first cohort of patients is allocated to dose x_1 with probability R_l calculated from the efficacy skeletons p_{kl}^* for each dose. In the proposed dose-finding method, toxicity and efficacy probabilities are estimated independently, but to provide a justifiable comparison to Hoering's method, Wages and Tait (2015) generated correlating binary outcomes using function **ranBin2** in **R** package **binarySimCLF**, that is, the log odds ratio specification used to generate the data was set to $\psi = 4.6$ to match that used by Hoering et al. (2013). Each simulation analyzed 1,000 trials.

To define the acceptable set, the maximum acceptable toxicity rate was specified to be $\phi_T = 0.33$, and the minimum efficacy threshold to be $\phi_E = 0.05$. The toxicity probabilities were modeled via the power model with skeleton values, which is robust and effective at carrying out the CRM designs. For efficacy, probabilities were modeled via the class of power models using 11 skeletons that correspond to the possible dose–efficacy relationship; six sets of values used for the unimodal relations, and five sets of values for plateau relations.

In all the scenarios, the mean of the recommended rates for true optimal dose of the proposed and Hoering's method were 73.9% and 57.7%, respectively. Under the scenarios that include one true optimal dose and where the dose–efficacy curves increase until the middle dose and remain constant after that dose—that is, the dose–efficacy curve nonmonotonically increases with the dose—the recommendation rates of the true optimal dose of the proposed method were higher than those of the Hoering's method by approximately 20–40%. In addition, the proposed method outperformed Hoering's method under the scenarios that include one true optimal dose and where the efficacy monotonically increases with the dose, by selection rates of approximately 10–40%.

Based on the results of simulation studies, regardless of whether the dose–response relationship of an investigational MTA is monotonic/nonmonotonic, the proposed method may show superior performance relative to Hoering's method.

4.2.4   Software Implementation

Readers can employ the dose-finding method proposed by Wages and Tait (2015) using the R code released at

http://faculty.virginia.edu/model-based_dose-finding/Wages%20and%20Tait%202015.R.

Wages and Tait (2015) provided two function pieces of code: **bpocrm** and **bpocrm.sim**. If we input the total number of doses, a set of toxicity skeleton values, the number of possible efficacy orderings, the possible efficacy orderings of the doses, the toxicity upper limit, efficacy lower limit, cohort size, the number of cohorts, starting dose, size of the adaptive randomization phase, the number of simulated trials, true toxicity probabilities, and true efficacy probabilities, then function **bpocrm.sim** outputs the operating characteristics of the method proposed by Wages and Tait (2015) as follows:

```
------------------------------------------------------------------
#####Specify the total number of doses
d<-5

###Specify a set of toxicity skeleton values
p.skel<-c(0.01,0.08,0.15,0.22,0.29)

#####Specify the number of possible efficacy orderings
g<-9    #efficacy

###Specify the possible efficacy orderings of the doses
 q.skel<-matrix(nrow=g,ncol=d)
 q.skel[1,]<-c(0.60,0.70,0.60,0.50,0.40)
 q.skel[2,]<-c(0.70,0.60,0.50,0.40,0.30)
 q.skel[3,]<-c(0.50,0.60,0.70,0.60,0.50)
 q.skel[4,]<-c(0.40,0.50,0.60,0.70,0.60)
 q.skel[5,]<-c(0.30,0.40,0.50,0.60,0.70)
 q.skel[6,]<-c(0.70,0.70,0.70,0.70,0.70)
 q.skel[7,]<-c(0.60,0.70,0.70,0.70,0.70)
 q.skel[8,]<-c(0.50,0.60,0.70,0.70,0.70)
 q.skel[9,]<-c(0.40,0.50,0.60,0.70,0.70)

tul<-0.33     ##toxicity upper limit
ell<-0.20     ##efficacy lower limit
cohortsize=1 ##cohort size for each inclusion
ncohort=48    ##number of cohorts
start.comb=1 ##starting dose
n.adaptive randomization=24        ##size of adaptive randomization phase
ntrial=1000   ##number of simulated trials
```

```
p0<-c(0.02,0.05,0.07,0.09,0.11)
q0<-c(0.68,0.56,0.49,0.40,0.33)
set.seed(580)     ##random seed

##simulate many trials
bpocrm.sim(p0,q0,p.skel,q.skel,tul,ell,cohortsize,ncohort,ntrial,
start.comb)
True tox probability:            0.02   0.05   0.07   0.09   0.11
True eff probability:            0.68   0.56   0.49   0.4    0.33
selection percentage:            69.7   21.0   8.4    0.7    0.2
number of toxicities:            0.4    0.5    0.5    0.4    0.3
number of responses:             15.4   5.9    3.5    1.8    1.0
number of patients treated:      22.6   10.5   7.0    4.6    3.2
percentage of stop (safety):      0
percentage of stop (futility):    0
```

4.3 The Dose-Finding Method Using the Change Point Model

Sato et al. (2016) developed an adaptive dose-finding method involving a change point logistic model to allow for more flexibility in modeling various dose–efficacy patterns (including the nonmonotonic pattern) for MTAs.

4.3.1 Modeling Toxicity and Efficacy Outcomes

Let Y_{Ei} and Y_{Ti} be binary efficacy and toxicity outcomes for the ith entering patient $(i = 1, \ldots, N)$, respectively. Y_{Ei} (or Y_{Ti}) $= 1$ indicates that efficacy (or toxicity) is observed, and Y_{Ei} (or Y_{Ti}) $= 0$ indicates otherwise.

To consider the correlation between the toxicity and efficacy outcomes, Sato et al. (2016) selected the model proposed by Islam et al. (2012). The joint probabilities for Y_{Ti} and Y_{Ei} are given in Table 4.1.

The bivariate joint probability function for Y_{Ei} and Y_{Ti} is expressed as

Table 4.1 The joint probabilities for Y_{Ei} and Y_{Ti}

		Y_{Ti}		
		0	1	
Y_{Ei}	0	π_{00}	π_{01}	$1 - \pi_E$
	1	π_{10}	π_{11}	π_E
		$1 - \pi_T$	π_T	1

$$\Pr(y_{Ei}, y_{Ti}) = \pi_{00}^{(1-y_{Ei})(1-y_{Ti})} \pi_{01}^{(1-y_{Ei})y_{Ti}} \pi_{10}^{y_{Ei}(1-y_{Ti})} \pi_{11}^{y_{Ei}y_{Ti}} = \prod_{j=0}^{1}\prod_{k=0}^{1} \pi_{jk}^{y_{ijk}}, \quad (4.11)$$

where

$$y_{i00} = (1 - y_{Ei})(1 - y_{Ti}), \quad j = 0, \ k = 0,$$
$$y_{i01} = (1 - y_{Ei})\, y_{Ti}, \quad j = 0, \ k = 1,$$
$$y_{i10} = y_{Ei}(1 - y_{Ti}), \quad j = 1, \ k = 0, \text{ and}$$
$$y_{i11} = y_{Ei}\, y_{Ti}, \quad j = 1, \ k = 1.$$

To model the probability of efficacy and toxicity outcomes, Eq. (4.11) is factorized into the conditional probability of toxicity given an efficacy outcome $\Pr(Y_{Ti} = k | Y_{Ei} = j; \ k, j = 0, 1)$ and the marginal probability of efficacy $\Pr(Y_{Ei} = j; \ j = 0, 1)$ as follows:

$$\Pr(y_{Ei}, y_{Ti}) = \prod_{j=0}^{1}\prod_{k=0}^{1} \pi_{jk}^{y_{ijk}} = \prod_{j=0}^{1}\prod_{k=0}^{1} \{\Pr(Y_{Ti} = k | Y_{Ei} = j)\Pr(Y_{Ei} = j)\}^{y_{ijk}}.$$

$$(4.12)$$

Sato et al. (2016) modeled the conditional probability functions of toxicity given each efficacy outcome using an ordinary logistic model, that is,

$$\Pr(Y_{Ti} = 1 | Y_{Ei} = 0) = \pi_{T|Y_E=0}(x_i; \theta_0) = \frac{\exp(\alpha_0 + \beta_0 x_i)}{1 + \exp(\alpha_0 + \beta_0 x_i)} \quad \text{and} \quad (4.13)$$

$$\Pr(Y_{Ti} = 1 | Y_{Ei} = 1) = \pi_{T|Y_E=1}(x_i; \theta_1) = \frac{\exp(\alpha_1 + \beta_1 x_i)}{1 + \exp(\alpha_1 + \beta_1 x_i)}, \quad (4.14)$$

where $x_i = \{d_1, \ldots, d_L\}$ is the actual dose of the agent administered to the ith patient, $\theta_0 = \{\alpha_0, \beta_0\}$ and $\theta_1 = \{\alpha_1, \beta_1\}$ are unknown parameters for the model of Eqs. (4.13) and (4.14), respectively. Given actual dose d_l $(l = 1, \ldots, L)$, the standardized dose is defined as $d'_l = \log(d_l) - L^{-1}\sum_{m=1}^{L} \log(d_m)$. It should be noted that these conditional models are equal (i.e., $\theta_0 = \theta_1$) at the independence of efficacy and toxicity (Islam et al. 2012).

Next, Sato et al. (2016) proposed the change point logistic model for marginal probability of efficacy as follows:

$$\Pr(Y_{Ei} = 1) = \pi_E(x_i) = \begin{cases} \pi_E(x_i; \theta_E) = \dfrac{\exp(\alpha_E + \beta_E x_i)}{1 + \exp(\alpha_E + \beta_E x_i)}, & x_i \leq d^* \\[4mm] \pi_E(x_i; \theta'_E) = \dfrac{\exp(\alpha'_E + \beta'_E x_i)}{1 + \exp(\alpha'_E + \beta'_E x_i)}, & x_i > d^* \end{cases}$$

$$(4.15)$$

where d^* is the change point of a dose between $d'_1, \ldots, d'_{L-1}$ and $\theta_E = \{\alpha_E, \beta_E\}$ and $\theta'_E = \{\alpha'_E, \beta'_E\}$ are unknown parameters.

For the current data on n patients, D_n, Sato et al. (2016) calculated the probabilities under the assumptions of $d^* = d'_1, \ldots, d'_{L-1}$, respectively, that is,

$$
\mathcal{L}_{n,l}\left(\theta_l | D_n, d^* = d'_l\right) = \prod_{i=1}^{n} \prod_{j=0}^{1} \prod_{k=0}^{1} \{\Pr\left(Y_{Ti} = k | Y_{Ei} = j\right) \Pr\left(Y_{Ei} = j\right)\}^{y_{ijk}}
$$

$$
= \prod_{i=1}^{n} \left\{\pi_{T|Y_E=0}\left(x_i; \theta_{0l}\right)\right\}^{y_{i01}} \left\{1 - \pi_{T|Y_E=0}\left(x_i; \theta_{0l}\right)\right\}^{y_{i00}}
$$

$$
\left\{\pi_{T|Y_E=1}\left(x_i; \theta_{1l}\right)\right\}^{y_{i11}} \left\{1 - \pi_{T|Y_E=1}\left(x_i; \theta_{1l}\right)\right\}^{y_{i10}}
$$

$$
\times \prod_{i \in \Omega} \left\{\pi_E\left(x_i; \theta_{El}\right)\right\}^{(y_{i11}+y_{i10})} \left\{1 - \pi_E\left(x_i; \theta_{El}\right)\right\}^{(y_{i00}+y_{i01})}
$$

$$
\times \prod_{i \notin \Omega} \left\{\pi_E\left(x_i; \theta'_{El}\right)\right\}^{(y_{i11}+y_{i10})} \left\{1 - \pi_E\left(x_i; \theta'_{El}\right)\right\}^{(y_{i00}+y_{i01})},
$$

$$(4.16)$$

where $\theta_l = \{\theta_{0l}, \theta_{1l}, \theta_{El}, \theta'_{El}\}$ and $\Omega = \{i | x_i \leq d^*, i = 1, \ldots, n\}$ is the set of patients who received a dose lower than the assumed change point of d^*. In the Bayesian inference for θ_l, Sato et al. (2016) assumed that the prior distribution for each parameter $f(\theta_l)$ is an independent normal distribution although other distributions can be used. The method for the specification of hyperparameters for a prior normal distribution will be described later.

For each $\mathcal{L}_{n,l}$ $(l = 1, \ldots, L - 1)$, the posterior distribution of θ_l is given by

$$
f\left(\theta_l | D_n, d^* = d'_l\right) \propto f(\theta_l) \mathcal{L}_{n,l}\left(\theta_l | D_n, d^* = d'_l\right). \tag{4.17}
$$

After calculating the posterior distributions of θ_l (for example, by Markov chain Monte Carlo methods), we can obtain the posterior mean $\hat{\theta}_l$ for each θ_l. The method for the specification of hyperparameters for a prior normal distribution is described in the next section.

Sato et al. (2016) devised a method for estimating change point (d^*) according to the method of Rukhin (1995). Given the posterior mean $\hat{\theta}_l$, we determine estimated change point $\tilde{d}^*$ that provides the maximum value among $\log \mathcal{L}_{n,l}\left(\hat{\theta}_l | D_n, d^* = d'_l\right)$, that is,

$$
\tilde{d}^* = \arg \max_{d'_1 \leq d^* \leq d'_{L-1}} \left\{\log \mathcal{L}_{n,l}\left(\hat{\theta}_l | D_n, d^* = d'_l\right)\right\}. \tag{4.18}
$$

Sato et al. (2016) proposed to estimate the value of the mean parameter via the prior probabilities of efficacy and toxicity outcomes for each dose that are often elicited from investigators. Let p_l be the prior probabilities of efficacy corresponding to dose d'_l. Given prior expected change point $d^{\#}$, the doses are categorized into two groups: $\{d'_l | d'_l \leq d^{\#}, l = 1, \ldots, L\}$ and $\{d'_l | d'_l > d^{\#}, l = 1, \ldots, L\}$. For the former and latter group, Sato et al. (2016) assumed $p_l = \exp\left(\eta_E + \xi_E d'_l\right) / \{1 + \exp\left(\eta_E + \xi_E d'_l\right)\}$ and $p_l = \exp\left(\eta'_E + \xi'_E d'_l\right) / \{1 + \exp\left(\eta'_E + \xi'_E d'_l\right)\}$ respectively, and then estimated $\theta_E = \{\eta_E, \xi_E\}$ and $\theta'_E = \{\eta'_E, \xi'_E\}$ by the least-squares method. Thus, the least-squares estimates of θ_E and θ'_E serve as the hyperparameter of prior normal distribution $\left(\text{i.e., } \alpha_E \sim Normal\left(\hat{\eta}_E, \sigma^2\right), \ \beta_E \sim Normal\left(\hat{\xi}_E, \sigma^2\right), \ \alpha'_E \sim Normal\left(\hat{\eta}'_E, \sigma^2\right), \ \text{and } \beta'_E \sim Normal\left(\hat{\xi}'_E, \sigma^2\right) \right)$.

To determine the mean parameter for each of the prior normal distributions for θ_0 and θ_1, Sato et al. (2016) first supposed that q_l are the prior probabilities of toxicity corresponding to dose d'_l. Sato et al. (2016) then introduced the conditional probabilities of toxicity given each efficacy outcome, $q_{T|Y_E=0, l}$ and $q_{T|Y_E=1, l}$, that can be written as p_l, q_l, and the prior correlation coefficient ψ_l, which is provided by Islam et al. (2012). For bivariate Bernoulli variables, the correlation coefficient is expressed as

$$\psi_l = \frac{\Pr\left(Y_E=1, Y_T=1, d'_l\right) \Pr\left(Y_E=0, Y_T=0, d'_l\right) - \Pr\left(Y_E=1, Y_T=0, d'_l\right) \Pr\left(Y_E=0, Y_T=1, d'_l\right)}{\sqrt{p_l\left(1-p_l\right) q_l\left(1-q_l\right)}}.$$

(4.19)

where

$$\Pr\left(Y_E=1, Y_T=1, d'_l\right) = q_l - q_{T|Y_E=0, l}\left(1-p_l\right) = q_{T|Y_E=1, l}\, p_l,$$
$$\Pr\left(Y_E=0, Y_T=0, d'_l\right) = \left(1-q_{T|Y_E=0, l}\right)\left(1-p_l\right) = 1 - q_l - \left(1-q_{T|Y_E=1, l}\right) p_l,$$
$$\Pr\left(Y_E=1, Y_T=0, d'_l\right) = 1 - q_l - \left(1-q_{T|Y_E=0, l}\right)\left(1-p_l\right) = \left(1-q_{T|Y_E=1, l}\right) p_l, \text{ and}$$
$$\Pr\left(Y_E=0, Y_T=1, d'_l\right) = q_{T|Y_E=0, l}\left(1-p_l\right) = q_l - q_{T|Y_E=1, l}\, p_l.$$

According to these equations, $q_{T|Y_E=0, l}$ and $q_{T|Y_E=1, l}$ can be expressed as

$$q_{T|Y_E=0, l} = \frac{\psi_l\sqrt{p_l\left(1-p_l\right) q_l\left(1-q_l\right)} - q_l\left(1-p_l\right)}{p_l - 1},$$

(4.20)

$$q_{T|Y_E=1, l} = \frac{\psi_l\sqrt{p_l\left(1-p_l\right) q_l\left(1-q_l\right)} + p_l q_l}{p_l}.$$

(4.21)

Thus, if we assume that $q_{T|Y_E=0, l} = \exp\left(\eta_0 + \xi_0 d'_l\right) / \left\{1 + \exp\left(\eta_0 + \xi_0 d'_l\right)\right\}$ and $q_{T|Y_E=1, l} = \exp\left(\eta_1 + \xi_1 d'_l\right) / \left\{1 + \exp\left(\eta_1 + \xi_1 d'_l\right)\right\}$, $\theta_0 = \{\eta_0, \xi_0\}$ and $\theta_1 = \{\eta_1, \xi_1\}$ are estimated by the least-squares method (i.e., $\alpha_0 \sim Normal\left(\hat{\eta}_0, \sigma^2\right)$, $\beta_0 \sim Normal\left(\hat{\xi}_0, \sigma^2\right)$, $\alpha_1 \sim Normal\left(\hat{\eta}_1, \sigma^2\right)$, and $\beta_1 \sim Normal\left(\hat{\xi}_1, \sigma^2\right)$).

In addition, the standard deviation (σ) is set to a common value for all the prior normal distributions in this study; however, it should be fine-tuned in a simulation study before the trial is conducted.

4.3.2 The Dose-Finding Algorithm

The Definition of the Optimal Dose:

Sato et al. (2016) defined an optimal dose as a dose level that has the minimum weighted Mahalanobis distance proposed by Hirakawa (2012). Sato et al. (2016) obtained the kth posterior samples of the weighted Mahalanobis distance of outcome

$\left(\pi_E^{(k)} \left(d_l' \right), \ \pi_T^{(k)} \left(d_l' \right) \right)$ to optimal point $(1, 0)$:

$$m^{(k)} \left(d_l' \right) = \sqrt{ \frac{ w_E^2 u_E \left(d_l' \right)^2 - 2\rho \left(d_l' \right) w_E w_T u_E \left(d_l' \right) u_T \left(d_l' \right) + w_T^2 u_T \left(d_l' \right)^2 }{ 1 - \rho \left(d_l' \right)^2 } }, \quad (4.22)$$

where

$$u_E \left(d_l' \right) = \frac{ 1 - \pi_E^{(k)} \left(d_l' \right) }{ \sqrt{ \pi_E^{(k)} \left(d_l' \right) \left\{ 1 - \pi_E^{(k)} \left(d_l' \right) \right\} } }, \quad (4.23)$$

$$u_T \left(d_l' \right) = \frac{ 0 - \pi_T^{(k)} \left(d_l' \right) }{ \sqrt{ \pi_T^{(k)} \left(d_l' \right) \left\{ 1 - \pi_T^{(k)} \left(d_l' \right) \right\} } }, \quad (4.24)$$

and w_E and w_T are the prespecified weight parameters for adjusting the trade-off between efficacy and toxicity, respectively. Suppose $\rho \left(d_l' \right)$ denotes the correlation coefficient (Islam et al. 2012):

$$\rho \left(d_l' \right) = \frac{ \pi_{11}^{(k)} \left(d_l' \right) \pi_{00}^{(k)} \left(d_l' \right) - \pi_{10}^{(k)} \left(d_l' \right) \pi_{01}^{(k)} \left(d_l' \right) }{ \sqrt{ \pi_E^{(k)} \left(d_l' \right) \left\{ 1 - \pi_E^{(k)} \left(d_l' \right) \right\} \pi_T^{(k)} \left(d_l' \right) \left\{ 1 - \pi_T^{(k)} \left(d_l' \right) \right\} } }, \quad (4.25)$$

where

$$\pi_{11}^{(k)} \left(d_l' \right) = \pi_T^{(k)} \left(d_l' \right) - \pi_{T|Y_E=0}^{(k)} \left(d_l' \right) \left\{ 1 - \pi_E^{(k)} \left(d_l' \right) \right\} = \pi_{T|Y_E=1}^{(k)} \left(d_l' \right) \pi_E^{(k)} \left(d_l' \right),$$

$$\pi_{00}^{(k)} \left(d_l' \right) = \left\{ 1 - \pi_{T|Y_E=0}^{(k)} \left(d_l' \right) \right\} \left\{ 1 - \pi_E^{(k)} \left(d_l' \right) \right\}$$
$$= 1 - \pi_T^{(k)} \left(d_l' \right) - \left\{ 1 - \pi_{T|Y_E=1}^{(k)} \left(d_l' \right) \right\} \pi_E^{(k)} \left(d_l' \right),$$

$$\pi_{10}^{(k)} \left(d_l' \right) = 1 - \pi_T^{(k)} \left(d_l' \right) - \left\{ 1 - \pi_{T|Y_E=0}^{(k)} \left(d_l' \right) \right\} \left\{ 1 - \pi_E^{(k)} \left(d_l' \right) \right\}$$
$$= \left\{ 1 - \pi_{T|Y_E=1}^{(k)} \left(d_l' \right) \right\} \pi_E^{(k)} \left(d_l' \right), \text{ and}$$

$$\pi_{01}^{(k)} \left(d_l' \right) = \pi_{T|Y_E=0}^{(k)} \left(d_l' \right) \left\{ 1 - \pi_E^{(k)} \left(d_l' \right) \right\} = \pi_T^{(k)} \left(d_l' \right) - \pi_{T|Y_E=1}^{(k)} \left(d_l' \right) \pi_E^{(k)} \left(d_l' \right).$$

The posterior mean of the weighted Mahalanobis distance is expressed as the average of the posterior samples, that is,

$$\bar{m} \left(d_l' \right) = \frac{1}{K} \sum_{k=1}^{K} m^{(k)} \left(d_l' \right). \quad (4.26)$$

In the simulation studies, Sato et al. (2016) ran 500 burn-in iterations and then recorded every 10th subsequent sample out of 10,000 Gibbs samples to reduce the autocorrelation in the Markov chain; accordingly, the value of K was set to 1,000 throughout.

Acceptable Dose Criteria:

To avoid allocating patients to ineffective or severely toxic doses, Sato et al. (2016) determined the set of acceptable doses (T) based on the posterior probabilities of efficacy and toxicity outcomes for each dose d'_l, $\hat{\pi}_E\left(d'_l\right)$ and $\hat{\pi}_T\left(d'_l\right)$ $\left(= \hat{\pi}_E\left(d'_l\right) \times \hat{\pi}_{T|Y_E=1}\left(d'_l\right) + \left\{1 - \hat{\pi}_E\left(d'_l\right)\right\} \times \hat{\pi}_{T|Y_E=0}\left(d'_l\right)\right)$, as follows (Thall and Cook 2004):

$$T\left(d'_l\right) = \left\{d'_l | \Pr\left\{\hat{\pi}_E\left(d'_l\right) > c_E\right\} > \delta_E \text{ and } \Pr\left\{\hat{\pi}_T\left(d'_l\right) < c_T\right\} > \delta_T, l = 1, \ldots, L\right\},$$
(4.27)

where c_E and c_T are critical values for the posterior probabilities of efficacy and toxicity outcomes, and δ_E and δ_T are fixed probability cutoffs, respectively. That is, Sato et al. (2016) extracted the doses that are expected to be effective and not very toxic at a certain level.

The Dose-Finding Algorithm:

To stabilize the parameter estimates for θ_l and d^* at an early stage of the trial, Sato et al. (2016) incorporated a run-in period wherein the first cohort of patients is treated with the lowest dose, and the dose is escalated unless two or more of three patients in that cohort experience toxicity, although other dose escalation rules, such as the well-known $3 + 3$ rule, can be applied. In this study, the cohort consisted of three patients.

Upon completion of the run-in period, the trial design switches to the model-based dose-finding stage. Using the estimated change point of $\tilde{d}^*$ and the corresponding posterior means of $\hat{\theta}_l$, Sato et al. (2016) calculated the posterior probabilities of efficacy and toxicity outcomes for each dose d'_l. The dose with the minimum value of $\bar{m}\left(d'_l\right)$ among $T\left(d'_l\right)$ is administered to the next cohort of patients. Sato et al. (2016) applied this algorithm until the maximum sample size was reached and then selected the dose administered to the next cohort of patients as the optimal dose. If there is no acceptable dose at an interim time point, then the trial is terminated at this time point, and no dose is selected as the optimal dose.

4.3.3 Operating Characteristics

Sato et al. (2016) compared the operating characteristics of the proposed method with the method proposed by Thall and Cook (2004) via simulations under 12 scenarios. In this simulation study, six actual doses were considered, and the maximum sample size was set to 36. The starting dose was set to the lowest dose, and the number of patients allocated to each dose level was set to 3. Sato et al. (2016) introduced a correlation between toxicity and efficacy into simulations by conditional probabilities $\Pr\left(Y_E = 1 | Y_T = 0, d_l'\right)$ and $\Pr\left(Y_E = 1 | Y_T = 1, d_l'\right)$, which were calculated by substituting true $\pi_T\left(d_l'\right)$, $\pi_E\left(d_l'\right)$, and $\rho\left(d_l'\right) = \rho = 0.20$ into the following equations:

$$\Pr\left(Y_E = 1 | Y_T = 0, d_l'\right) = \frac{\rho\sqrt{\pi_E\left(d_l'\right)\left\{1 - \pi_E\left(d_l'\right)\right\}\pi_T\left(d_l'\right)\left\{1 - \pi_T\left(d_l'\right)\right\}} - \pi_E\left(d_l'\right)\left\{1 - \pi_T\left(d_l'\right)\right\}}{\pi_T\left(d_l'\right) - 1},$$

(4.28)

$$\Pr\left(Y_E = 1 | Y_T = 1, d_l'\right) = \frac{\rho\sqrt{\pi_E\left(d_l'\right)\left\{1 - \pi_E\left(d_l'\right)\right\}\pi_T\left(d_l'\right)\left\{1 - \pi_T\left(d_l'\right)\right\}} + \pi_E\left(d_l'\right)\pi_T\left(d_l'\right)}{\pi_T\left(d_l'\right)}.$$

(4.29)

Each simulation consisted of 1,000 trials.

The critical values for the posterior probabilities of efficacy and toxicity c_E and c_T were set to 0.20 and 0.40, respectively, and fixed probability cutoffs δ_E and δ_T were both set to 0.10. To determine the mean of the prior normal distribution in the proposed method, Sato et al. (2016) specified the prior efficacy and toxicity probabilities as $(p_1, p_2, p_3, p_4, p_5, p_6) = (0.05, 0.20, 0.35, 0.50, 0.55, 0.60)$ and $(q_1, q_2, q_3, q_4, q_5, q_6) = (0.05, 0.10, 0.15, 0.20, 0.25, 0.30)$, respectively. The expected change point was set to $d^\# = d_4'$, the correlation coefficient of $\psi_l = \psi = 0.20$, and the standard deviation of $\sigma = 3.0$. The weight parameters w_E and w_T for the weighted Mahalanobis distance were set to 1.0.

Throughout the 11 scenarios, which include a true optimal dose, the means of the recommended rates for the true optimal dose of the proposed method and of Thall and Cook's method were 44.1% and 26.8%, respectively. In the scenarios where the dose–efficacy curve nonmonotonically increases with the dose, the recommendation rates for the optimal dose and the average number of patients allocated to the optimal dose in the proposed method were up to 40% higher as compared with Thall and Cook's method. This index of the proposed method was not worse than that of Thall and Cook's method under the scenarios where the dose–efficacy curve monotonically increases with the dose level. Under the scenarios where the optimal dose was located at the lowest (or highest) dose level, the two methods were comparable. In the case where all dose levels had unacceptable toxicity, the two methods yielded an approximately 100% termination rate of the trial.

The simulation studies indicated that the operating characteristics in the proposed method were more favorable than those of the Thall and Cook method, especially when the optimal dose levels were in the lower or middle range, and the dose–efficacy curves nonmonotonically increased with the dose escalation. Thus, the proposed method may be useful for determining the optimal dose in the cases where the MTAs under study have a nonmonotonic dose–efficacy relationship according to prior information, such as preclinical data.

4.3.4 Software Implementation

The estimation of model parameters under the assumptions of change point $d^* = d'_1, \ldots, d'_{L-1}$ is carried out by means of PROC MCMC in SAS, version 9.3 (SAS Institute Inc., Cary, NC). Given the prior distribution for each parameter and the assumed change point $d^* = d'_l$, the following programs apply the random-walk Metropolis algorithm for input SAS dataset "assign" and output posterior mean $\hat{\theta}_l$ at the assumed change point. Dataset "assign" contains a dose for patient i, y_{i00}, y_{i01}, y_{i10}, and y_{i11}.

```
----------------------------------------------------
/************************************************/
D: actual dose
X: standardized dose calculated based on actual dose
Y00: no efficacy and no toxicity outcome
Y01: no efficacy and toxicity outcome
Y10: efficacy and no toxicity outcome
Y11: efficacy and toxicity outcome
CHANGEPOINT: assumptive change-point
/************************************************/

PROC MCMC DATA=assign NTU=&NTU. NBI=&NBI. NMC=&NMC.
                  NTHIN=&NTHIN. PROPCOV=QUANEW SEED=&SEED.
                  OUTPOST=OUT;

    ODS OUTPUT POSTSUMMARIES=OUT_SUMMARIES;

    ***** Parameter definition *****;
    PARMS ALPHACT0;
    PARMS ALPHACT1;
    ARRAY ALPHAE[2];
    PARMS (ALPHAE1 ALPHAE2);

    PARMS BETACT0;
    PARMS BETACT1;
    ARRAY BETAE[2];
    PARMS (BETAE1 BETAE2);
    ******************************;

    ***** Prior distribution ****************;
    PRIOR ALPHACT1 ~ NORMAL(-0.951,SD=3);
    PRIOR ALPHACT0 ~ NORMAL(-2.191,SD=3);
    PRIOR ALPHAE1 ~ NORMAL(-0.599,SD=3);
    PRIOR ALPHAE2 ~ NORMAL(-0.375,SD=3);

    PRIOR BETACT1 ~ NORMAL(0.353, SD=3);
    PRIOR BETACT0 ~ NORMAL(0.936, SD=3);
    PRIOR BETAE1 ~ NORMAL(2.114, SD=3);
    PRIOR BETAE2 ~ NORMAL(1.123, SD=3);
    *****************************************;

    *****  Conditional toxicity probability *****;
    PCT0=LOGISTIC(ALPHACT0+BETACT0*X);
    PCT1=LOGISTIC(ALPHACT1+BETACT1*X);
    *********************************************;
```

```
***** Change-point Model **************;
J = 1 + (D > &CHANGEPOINT.);
PE=LOGISTIC(ALPHAE[J] + BETAE[J]*X);
******************************************;

LLIKE=Y01*LOG(PCT0)+Y00*LOG(1-PCT0)
         +Y11*LOG(PCT1)+Y10*LOG(1-PCT1)
         +(Y11+Y10)*LOG(PE)+(Y00+Y01)*LOG(1-PE);
MODEL DGENERAL(LLIKE);

RUN;
----------------------------------------------------
```

4.4 The Dose-Finding Method with Late-Onset Efficacy

Riviere et al. (2016) proposed a dose-finding method for MTAs with efficacy delayed
so often that the efficacy practically takes more follow-up time to assess as compared
with toxicity. Riviere et al. (2016) employed a logistic model with a plateau parameter
to consider the plateau dose–efficacy relationship for MTAs.

4.4.1 Modeling Toxicity and Efficacy Outcomes

Let us assume that Y_i is the binary toxicity outcome for patient i ($i = 1, \ldots, N$).
$Y_i = 1$ indicates that toxicity is observed, and $Y_i = 0$ indicates otherwise. To consider
late-onset efficacy, let T be a fixed time window required to evaluate efficacy, and
t_{Ei} denotes time to efficacy of the ith patient. Suppose C_{Ei} is the follow-up time
for patient i prior to the entry of the next patient. The efficacy indicator of patient
i prior to the entry of the next patient is denoted by $z_i = I[t_{Ei} < C_{Ei}]$, where $I[\cdot]$
represents the indicator function.

Riviere et al. (2016) modeled the toxicity probability of dose d_l ($l = 1, \ldots, L$),
designated as $\pi_T(d_l) = \pi_{Tl}$, via a logistic model:

$$\text{logit}(\pi_{Tl}) = \beta_0 + \beta_1 u_l, \tag{4.30}$$

where β_0, $\beta_1(> 0)$ are unknown parameters, and u_l is the effective dose associated
with dose d_l, which typically differs from the actual dose. To make u_l identifiable, we
require the prior estimates of $\tilde{\beta}_0$, $\tilde{\beta}_1$, and $\tilde{\pi}_{Tl}$. Then, effective dose u_l is determined
by back-solving the dose–toxicity model as follows,

$$u_l = \left\{ \log\left(\frac{\tilde{\pi}_{Tl}}{1 - \tilde{\pi}_{Tl}}\right) - \tilde{\beta}_0 \right\} / \tilde{\beta}_1.$$

Next, let $\pi_E(d_l) = \pi_{El}$ be the efficacy probability for dose d_l. Riviere et al. (2016) employed a logistic model with plateau parameter τ to capture the increasing-then-plateauing feature of the dose–efficacy relationship:

$$\text{logit}(\pi_{El}) = \gamma_0 + \gamma_1 (v_l \, I \, [d_l < \tau] + v_\tau \, I \, [d_l \geq \tau]) \tag{4.31}$$

where γ_0 and γ_1 are unknown parameters, and v_l is the effective dose associated with dose d_l. Plateau parameter τ is an integer between 1 and L that indicates at which dose level the dose–efficacy curve reaches the plateau. Like effective dose u_l, v_l is determined by back-solving the dose–efficacy model as follows:

$$v_l = \left\{ \log \left(\frac{\tilde{\pi}_{El}}{1 - \tilde{\pi}_{El}} \right) - \tilde{\gamma}_0 \right\} / \tilde{\gamma}_1,$$

where $\tilde{\pi}_{El}$, $\tilde{\gamma}_0$, $\tilde{\gamma}_1$ and $\tilde{\tau}$ are prior estimates of parameters.

After the first n patients are enrolled into the trial, the likelihood of toxicity data D_{tox} is

$$\mathcal{L}(\beta_0, \beta_1 | D_{tox}) = \prod_{i=1}^{n} \pi_{Tx_i}^{y_i} \left(1 - \pi_{Tx_i} \right)^{1-y_i}, \tag{4.32}$$

where x_i denotes the effective dose corresponding to the actual dose administered to the ith patient.

If we assume that $f(\beta_0, \beta_1)$ represents the prior distribution of β_0 and β_1, the posterior is then given by

$$f(\beta_0, \beta_1 | D_{tox}) \, \mathcal{L}(\beta_0, \beta_1 | D_{tox}) \, f(\beta_0, \beta_1). \tag{4.33}$$

Riviere et al. (2016) assumed that prior distributions are independent and take a vague normal prior $N(0, 100)$ for the intercept β_0, and we assigned slope β_1 to an exponential distribution with a rate parameter of 1, i.e., $\beta_1 \approx Exp(1)$. After we specify the prior distributions, the posterior distribution is sampled using the Gibbs sampler.

For efficacy, Riviere et al. (2016) followed the approach of Cheung and Chappell (2000) by weighting the observed data likelihood with the follow-up time. Given efficacy data D_{eff}, the weighted likelihood function of the efficacy data is expressed as

$$\mathcal{L}(\gamma_0, \gamma_1, \tau | D_{eff}) = \prod_{i=1}^{n} \left(w_i \pi_{Ex_i} \right)^{z_i} \left(1 - w_i \pi_{Ex_i} \right)^{1-z_i} \tag{4.34}$$

where w_i is the weight function.

Riviere et al. (2016) selected the form of adaptive weights proposed by Cheung and Thall (2002), formulated as

$$w_i = \begin{cases} 1 & \text{if } t_{Ei} \leq C_{Ei} \\ \dfrac{\#\{j \, : \, t_{Ej} \leq C_{Ei} \text{ and } C_{Ej}=T\}+C_{Ei}/T}{\#\{j \, : \, t_{Ej} \leq T \text{ and } C_{Ej}=T\}+1} & otherwise \end{cases} \tag{4.35}$$

where $\#\{j \, : \, t_{Ej} \leq T \text{ and } C_{Ej} = T\}$ is the number of patients who experienced efficacy (i.e., $t_{Ej} \leq T$) and completed the follow-up (i.e., $C_{Ej} = T$) before the entry of the next patient; and C_{Ei}/T is the proportion of the time that patient i was followed compared to the full follow-up time T before the entry of the next patient.

If we assume that $f(\gamma_0, \gamma_1, \tau)$ represents the prior distribution of γ_0, γ_1, and τ, then the posterior is given by

$$f(\gamma_0, \gamma_1, \tau | D_{eff}) \propto \mathcal{L}(\gamma_0, \gamma_1, \tau | D_{eff}) f(\gamma_0, \gamma_1, \tau). \tag{4.36}$$

Riviere et al. (2016) assumed that prior distributions are independent and took vague normal prior $N(0, 100)$ for the intercept γ_0 and an exponential distribution with a rate parameter of 1 for γ_1, i.e., $\gamma_1 \approx Exp(1)$. To the plateau parameter, τ, Riviere et al. (2016) assigned a discrete prior distribution $\Pr(\tau = l) = p_l$ and $\sum_{m=1}^{L} p_m = 1$ and $\forall m, p_m \geq 0$. When no information is available on the plateau location, the uniform prior is recommended with $p_1 = \cdots = p_L = 1/L$. After we specified the prior distributions, the posterior distribution is sampled by the Gibbs sampler.

4.4.2 Plateau Estimation

With the Gibbs sampler, the posterior probability of the lth dose being the plateau point, $q_l = \Pr(\tau = d_l | D_{eff})$, is given by

$$q_l = \frac{p_l \int \int \mathcal{L}(\gamma_0, \gamma_1 | d_l, D_{eff}) f(\gamma_0, \gamma_1) d\gamma_1 d\gamma_0}{\sum_{m=1}^{L} p_m \int \int \mathcal{L}(\gamma_0, \gamma_1 | d_m, D_{eff}) f(\gamma_0, \gamma_1) d\gamma_1 d\gamma_0}. \tag{4.37}$$

Riviere et al. (2016) proposed two approaches to plateau estimation:

MTA-RA (Adaptive Randomization):

Let us assume that R is the set of doses whose posterior probabilities of being the plateau point were close to the largest one with a difference less than a positive threshold s_1, i.e.,

$$R = \left\{ k \, : \, \left| \max_{1 \leq l \leq L} (q_l) - q_k \right| \leq s_1, 1 \leq k \leq L \right\}, \tag{4.38}$$

where s_1 is the cutoff value. Riviere et al. (2016) found that what generally works well in their simulation study is $s_1 = 0.20 \left(1 - \frac{n}{N}\right)$, where n is the current sample size. The plateau estimate, $\hat{\tau}$, is sampled from R with renormalized probability $q_l / \sum_{k \in R} q_k$.

MTA-PM (Posterior Efficacy Probabilities):

Given the plateau location at each possible dose level and estimated posterior efficacy probabilities, we then perform BMA on the estimated posterior efficacy probabilities

$$\bar{\pi}_{El} = \sum_{k=1}^{L} \hat{\pi}_E (d_l, \gamma_0, \gamma_1 | \tau = k) q_k \tag{4.39}$$

where $\hat{\pi}_E (d_l, \gamma_0, \gamma_1 | \tau = k)$ is the posterior mean of the efficacy probability under the assumption that $\tau = k$. After that, the plateau is determined at dose

$$\hat{\tau} = \max \left\{ k \; : \; 1 \leq k \leq L, \; \bar{\pi}_{Ek} - \bar{\pi}_{E(k-1)} \geq s_2 \right\} \tag{4.40}$$

where s_2 is a cutoff value. The value of s_2, which is a constant, should be calibrated in a simulation to ensure good operating characteristics of the design.

4.4.3   The Dose-Finding Algorithm

Definition of the Optimal Dose:

Riviere et al. (2016) defined the optimal dose as the dose level that has the maximum efficacy probability among the admissible dose levels.

Acceptable Dose Criteria:

Riviere et al. (2016) regarded the dose that satisfies the following safety and efficacy requirements as admissible:

$$\Pr (\pi_{Tl} > \theta) < L_T \tag{4.41}$$

$$\Pr (\pi_{El} > \xi) \geq L_E \; I \; [n_k > \max (c, 3)] \tag{4.42}$$

where θ and ξ are the prespecified toxicity upper bound and efficacy lower bound, L_T and L_E are the respective probability thresholds for toxicity and efficacy, and n_k denotes the number of patients treated with dose d_l, respectively. Here, the set of admissible doses that met the two above-mentioned criteria is designated as $A (d_l)$.

The Dose-Finding Algorithm:

At the beginning of the trial, the following start-up phase is implemented to gather enough information for estimating model parameters. The first cohort of patients is at the lowest dose level 1, and the dose is escalated to the next dose level unless more than one out of three patients in that cohort experiences toxicity.

Once a toxicity is observed or the highest dose level is reached, the start-up phase ends, and the trial design switches to the model-based dose-finding phase, where patients are treated at a cohort size of c. The next incoming cohort of patients is basically assigned to the dose level with the highest efficacy in the set of admissible doses $A(d_l)$:

$$d^{next} = \min\left(\arg\max_{l \in A(d_l)}\left(\hat{\pi}_{El}\right)\right) \tag{4.43}$$

If d^{next} is the dose that has never been administered up to that time point, increasing the dose by only one level, Riviere et al. (2016) continued the above dose assignment processes until the maximum sample size was reached, and selected the optimal dose as the lowest dose level that is admissible and has the highest estimate of efficacy among all the doses tested during the trial. At any time during the model-based dose-finding phase, if all doses were not admissible, those authors terminated the trial to protect patients from overly toxic or futile doses.

4.4.4 Operating Characteristics

Riviere et al. (2016) compared the proposed MTA-RA and MTA-PM designs with the method proposed by Hunsberger et al. (2005) (abbreviated as the HRDK method) and the method proposed by Thall and Cook (2004) (abbreviated as the TC method) under 10 scenarios. Because the HRDK and TC designs assume that the efficacy endpoint is binary, it is quickly ascertainable when these two designs are implemented. Riviere et al. (2016) assumed six dose levels, and the maximum sample size was $N = 60$. The trial started at the lowest dose d_1, and the cohort size was $c = 3$ patients. They considered toxicity and efficacy independent. Each simulation was conducted 2,000 times.

Riviere et al. (2016) set the prespecified toxicity upper bound as $\theta = 0.35$, the toxicity threshold as $L_T = 0.90$, the efficacy lower bound as $\xi = 0.20$, and the efficacy threshold as $L_E = 0.40$. To identify effective doses u_k and v_k used in the toxicity and efficacy models, Riviere et al. (2016) took the initial guesses of toxicity and efficacy probabilities as (0.02, 0.06, 0.12, 0.20, 0.30, 0.40) and (0.12, 0.20, 0.30, 0.40, 0.50, 0.59), respectively. The patient accrual followed a Poisson process at the rate of 0.28 patients per week. The evaluation of efficacy required 7 weeks. Riviere et al. (2016) assumed that the time to efficacy followed an exponential distribution whose parameter was chosen based on the efficacy rate of each dose under each scenario. It should be noted that when implementing the HRDK and TC method, Riviere et al. (2016) waited for the efficacy response of the treated patients to become completely observable before enrolling a new cohort of patients.

In the scenarios that include a true optimal dose, the means of the recommended rates for the true optimal dose of MTA-RA, MTA-PM, HRDK, and TC methods were 52.2%, 52.7%, 28.0%, and 34.7%, respectively. Although the TC method performed the best under the scenario where the plateau was reached at the lowest dose level (the differences in the probabilities of correct optimal dose selection between their proposed method and TC method were approximately 10%), their proposed method outperformed the HRDK design and performed as well as or better than TC in terms of the selection of the optimal dose under most scenarios. In the scenario in which none of the doses was admissible and the trial had to be terminated, their proposed method terminated the trial early approximately 90% of the time.

In this simulation study, their method was based on partial information, while all patients' outcomes were fully determined in the other methods. Considering these simulation results, their proposed methods may outperform other dose-finding methods even in the case where efficacy takes a relatively long time to assess as compared to toxicity.

4.4.5 Software Implementation

Readers can employ the dose-finding method proposed by Riviere et al. (2016) using the **R** package **dfmta**.

Given the number of dose levels, the true toxicity probabilities, the true efficacy probabilities, toxicity upper bound, efficacy lower bound, initial guesses of toxicity probabilities, initial guesses of efficacy probabilities, the rate for the Poisson process used to simulate patient arrival, the total number of patients, cohort size for the start-up phase, cohort size for the model phase, the type of outcome for efficacy (time to event or binary), the method for plateau determination, s_1 (or s_2), the number of simulations, an toxicity threshold, and an efficacy threshold, function **mtaBin_sim** provides the operating characteristics of the method proposed by Riviere et al. (2016) as follows:

```
----------------------------------------------------------------
p_tox_sc1 = c(0.005, 0.01, 0.02, 0.05, 0.10, 0.15)
p_eff_sc1_g1 = c(0.01, 0.10, 0.30, 0.50, 0.80, 0.80)
p_tox_sc2 = c(0.01, 0.05, 0.10, 0.25, 0.50, 0.70)
p_eff_sc2_g2 = matrix(c(0.40, 0.01, 0.40, 0.02, 0.40, 0.05, 0.40,
0.10, 0.40, 0.35, 0.40, 0.55), nrow=2)
prior_tox = c(0.02, 0.06, 0.12, 0.20, 0.30, 0.40)
prior_eff = c(0.12, 0.20, 0.30, 0.40, 0.50, 0.59)
prior_eff2 = rbind(prior_eff, prior_eff)
s_1=function(n_cur){0.2}
n=60

sim = mtaBin_sim(ndose=6, p_tox= p_tox_sc1, p_eff= p_eff_sc1_g1,
tox_max=0.35, eff_min=0.20, prior_tox=prior_tox, prior_eff= prior_eff,
poisson_rate=0.28, n=60, cohort_start=3, cohort=3, tite=FALSE,
method="MTA-RA", s_1= function(n_cur){0.2*(1-n_cur/n)}, nsim=1,
c_tox=0.90, c_eff=0.40)
|----|----|----|----|----|----|----|----|----|----|
***************************************************|
> sim
Call:
mtaBin_sim(ngroups = 1, ndose = 6, p_tox = p_tox_sc1,
p_eff = p_eff_sc1_g1, tox_max = 0.35, eff_min = 0.2,
```

```
prior_tox = prior_tox, prior_eff = prior_eff, n = n,
cohort_start = 3, cohort = 3, tite = FALSE, method = "MTA-RA",
s_1 = function(n_cur) {0.2 * (1 - n_cur/n)}, nsim = 1)
doses
1 2 3 4 5 6
True toxicities 0.00 0.01 0.02 0.05 0.1 0.15
True efficacies for group 1 0.01 0.10 0.30 0.50 0.8 0.80
Prior toxicities 0.02 0.06 0.12 0.20 0.3 0.40
Prior efficacies for group 1 0.12 0.20 0.30 0.40 0.5 0.59
Percentage of Selection for group 1 0.00 0.00 0.00 0.00 0.0 100.00
Number of patients for group 1 3.00 3.00 3.00 6.00 6.0 39.00
Number of toxicities for group 1 0.00 0.00 0.00 0.00 0.0 10.00
Number of efficacies for group 1 0.00 1.00 1.00 2.00 5.0 33.00

Percentage of inconclusive trials for group 1: 0
Allocation method: MTA-RA
Number of simulations: 1
Total patients accrued: 60
Toxicity upper bound: 0.35
Efficacy lower bound: 0.2
Patient arrival for group 1 is modeled as a Poisson process with rate:
1 that is in mean 1 patients during a full follow-up time
Toxicity threshold: 0.9
Efficacy threshold: 0.4
Cohort size start-up phase: 3
Cohort size model phase: 3
Efficiency is not a time-to-event but binary
------------------------------------------------------------------
```

References

Cai, C., Yuan, Y., Ji, Y.: A Bayesian dose finding design for oncology clinical trials of combinational biological agents. Appl. Stat. **63**, 159–173 (2014)

Cheung, Y.K., Chappell, R.: Sequential designs for phase I clinical trials with late-onset toxicities. Biometrics **56**, 1177–1182 (2000)

Cheung, Y.K., Thall, P.F.: Monitoring the rates of composite events with censored data in phase II clinical trials. Biometrics **58**, 89–97 (2002)

Fox, E., Curt, G., Balis, F.: Clinical trial design for target-based therapy. Oncologist **7**, 401–409 (2002)

Hirakawa, A.: An adaptive dose-finding approach for correlated bivariate binary and continuous outcomes in phase I oncology trials. Stat. Med. **31**, 516–532 (2012)

Hoering, A., Mitchell, A., LeBlanc, M., Crowley, J.: Early phase trial design for assessing several dose levels for toxicity and efficacy for targeted agents. Clin. Trials **10**, 422–429 (2013)

Hunsberger, S., Rubinstein, L.V., Dancey, J., Korn, E.L.: Dose escalation trial designs based on a molecularly targeted endpoint. Stat. Med. **24**, 2171–2181 (2005)

Islam, M.A., Chowdhury, R.I., Briollais, L.: A bivariate binary model for testing dependence in outcomes. Bull. Malays. Math. Sci. Soc. **35**, 845–858 (2012)

Le Tourneau, C., Dieras, V., Tresca, P., Cacheux, W., Paoletti, X.: Current challenges for the early clinical development of anticancer drugs in the era of molecularly targeted agents. Target Oncol. **5**, 65–72 (2015)

Riviere, M.K., Yuan, Y., Dubois, F., Zohar, S.: A Bayesian dose finding design for clinical trials combining a cytotoxic agent with a molecularly targeted agent. Appl. Stat. **64**, 215–229 (2015)

Riviere, M.K., Yuan, Y., Jourdan, J.H., Dubois, F., Zohar, S.: Phase I/II dose-finding design for molecularly targeted agent: plateau determination using adaptive randomization. Stat. Methods Med. Res. (2016). https://doi.org/10.1177/0962280216631763

Rukhin, A.L.: Asymptotic behavior of estimators of the change-point in a binomial probability. J. Appl. Stat. Sci. **1**, 1–12 (1995)

Sato, H., Hirakawa, A., Hamada, C.: An adaptive dose-finding method using a change-point model for molecularly targeted agents in phase I trials. Stat. Med. **35**, 4093–4109 (2016)

Thall, P.F., Cook, J.D.: Dose-finding based on efficacy-toxicity trade-offs. Biometrics **60**, 684–693 (2004)

Wages, N.A., Tait, C.: Seamless phase I/II adaptive design for oncology trials of molecularly targeted agents. J. Biopharm. Stat. **25**, 903–920 (2015)

Chapter 5
Advanced Topics on Dose-Finding Designs

Abstract Recently, many types of dose-finding methods were proposed to address the issues that we often encounter in practice. For instance, a seamless phase I/II trial that combines phase I and phase II trials has some advantages: the data on both toxicity and efficacy can be used more efficiently for identifying an RP2D, and the duration of drug development can be reduced. For some MTAs, toxicity and efficacy outcomes sometimes require a longer follow-up period for their final assessments in practice. Moreover, there are patients who experience chronic low-grade toxicities from MTAs during the evaluation period of phase I trials. Such events eventually warrant a dose reduction or treatment interruption owing to intolerance. The relative dose intensity, which is generally defined as the ratio of the effectively delivered dose to the theoretically administered cumulative dose, draws the attention as a potential new endpoint of phase I trials. Cancer immunotherapy and dose individualization for phase I trials that analyze the mutations in several genes are also discussed.

Keywords Dose individualization · Immunotherapy · Phase I/II
Relative dose intensity

5.1 Leveraging Phase I/II Trials

The standard approach to early exploratory clinical trials for developing new drugs in oncology is to conduct phase I and phase II trials separately, where an MTD is determined in phase I trials, and the efficacy at the MTD is assessed in phase II trials. This approach has also been applied to the development of drug combinations. An alternative approach is to combine these trials, so that the data on both toxicity and efficacy can be used more efficiently for identifying an optimal dose, and the duration of drug development can be reduced. For example, Hoering et al. (2011) proposed a two-step dose-finding trial for assessing both toxicity and efficacy of a target agent. A traditional dose-finding design is employed at the first step. At this step, only toxicity is assessed, and the MTD is determined. For the second step, Hoering et al. (2011) proposed a modified phase II selection design for two or three dose levels at

© The Author(s), under exclusive licence to Springer Japan KK, part of Springer Nature 2018   81
A. Hirakawa et al., *Modern Dose-Finding Designs for Cancer Phase I Trials:*
Drug Combinations and Molecularly Targeted Agents, JSS Research Series
in Statistics, https://doi.org/10.1007/978-4-431-55573-5_5

and below the MTD to determine efficacy and to evaluate the efficacy and toxicity of each dose level.

In two-agent combination trials, it may also be reasonable to determine the RP2D on the basis of efficacy and toxicity outcomes by conducting a seamless phase I/II trial. Such trials generally involve determination of a single MTD combination based solely on toxicity data as a phase I part, followed by evaluation of efficacy data (such as response rates) at the MTD of the combination as a phase II part. Some dose-finding methods have been developed for determining an optimal-dose combination of two agents more efficiently based on toxicity and efficacy data in phase I/II trials (Table 5.1).

Huang et al. (2007) proposed to select a set of dose combinations with admissible toxicity using the $3 + 3$ design as the phase I part and to determine an optimal-dose combination based on efficacy data among the selected dose combinations via adaptive randomization as the phase II part. Yuan and Yin (2011a) proposed to employ a Bayesian copula-type model to select admissible toxicity dose combinations in the phase I part. In these methods, the evaluation of efficacy in the phase II part is restricted to a few selected dose combinations from the phase I part, but they do not necessarily include the true optimal-dose combination because of being based only on toxicity profiles from small numbers of patients in the phase I part. Wages and Conaway (2014) proposed adaptive randomization based on efficacy data among admissible toxicity dose combinations for patient allocation in the phase I part and then to determine an optimal-dose combination judging by the maximum estimated efficacy probability in the phase II part. Shimamura et al. (in press) proposed a zone-finding stage that determines the most admissible toxicity zone in the dose combination matrix and subsequently to select the dose combination allocated to the next patient from that zone in phase I.

5.2 Late-Onset Toxicity and Efficacy Outcomes

In practice, toxicity and efficacy outcomes sometimes require a longer follow-up period for their final assessments. According to Muler et al. (2004), it took 9 weeks to conduct follow-up for final evaluation of toxicities in the phase I trials of combined cisplatin and gemcitabine in patients with pancreatic cancer. Such late-onset outcomes cause logistical issues for implementation of the dose-finding method because it is undesirable to delay a new patient's treatment until the final evaluations of toxicity and/or efficacy outcomes of the previously enrolled patients in the trial are obtained. The issue of late-onset toxicity should be adequately addressed in the emerging era of MTAs. A review paper that examined the time-to-toxicity onset of MTAs revealed that 57% of grade 3 and 4 toxicities have a late onset (Postel-Vinay et al. 2011). To address the issue of late-onset toxicity, Cheung and Chappell (2000) proposed the time-to-event CRM that assigns weights to the responses of patients whose final response status has not been determined in single-agent trials. Mauguen et al. (2011) extended this weighting approach to the escalation with

Table 5.1 Phase I/II dose-finding design for two-agent combination trials

Method	Phase I/II dose-finding design for two-agent combinations using fixed-reference adaptive randomization	Phase I/II dose-finding design for two-agent combinations using Bayesian moving-reference adaptive randomization	Dose-finding design for two-agent combinations assuming partially ordered dose–toxicity and dose–efficacy relationships	Two-stage design based on zone and dose findings for two-agent combination phase I/II trials
Reference	Huang et al. (2007)	Yuan and Yin (2011a)	Wages and Conaway (2014)	Shimamura et al. (in press)
Model for toxicity	n/a	Copula-type model	Power model	Logistic model
Model for efficacy	Logistic model	Bayesian hierarchical model	Power model	Logistic model
Stage 1 dose-finding algorithm	1. The dose combinations are divided into zone along a diagonal of the dose combination matrix $D = (d_{ab})$; the first zone has a single combination dose d_{11}, and the second zone has two combination dose d_{12} and so on 2. The zone escalation starts with the first zone, and follows with the second zone, and then third zone, and so on 3. Modified '3 + 3' design based on the toxicity outcome is used for zone escalation 4. Dose combinations in the same zone are tested simultaneously using blocked randomization to control the number of patients for each dose combination	1. The posterior estimates of toxicity probabilities are estimated based on the Bayesian theorem 2. The next cohort of patients is allocated to the dose combination having toxicity closest to the target toxicity probability. One dose level of change only and not allowing a simultaneous escalation or de-escalation of both agents 3. Unless stopping criteria are met, this dose-finding step is continued until the prespecified sample size is reached	1. For toxicity and efficacy, some class of partial ordering is considered, respectively 2. The ordering probabilities that represent the relative certainty for each ordering are prespecified based on prior information. These probabilities are adaptively updated as posterior probabilities based on Bayesian theorem 3. When a new patient is to be enrolled, single ordering is selected with the largest posterior ordering probability 4. In the Bayesian framework, the posterior mean of toxicity and efficacy are generated for selected ordering 5. The admissible dose combinations are chosen based on the estimated toxicity probabilities 6. On the basis of the estimated efficacy probabilities for combinations in the admissible dose combinations, a randomization probability is calculated 7. The next cohort of patients is randomized to the combination with this probability 8. Unless stopping criteria are met, this dose-finding step is continued until the prespecified sample size is reached	1. Based on the partial ordering of toxicity probability, the dose combination matrix is categorized into the several zones which include the dose combination with unknown ordering of true toxicity probability 2. The toxicity probability for each zone is modeled by the power model and estimated based on Bayesian theorem 3. The first patient is treated with the lowest dose combination in first zone 4. Given the allocated zone and the toxicity outcome obtained for each patient at this time point, the toxicity probability for each zone is estimated, and then the single zone that has toxicity closest to the target toxicity probability is selected 5. The next cohort of patients is allocated to the dose combination with the least number of patients in the selected zone. If there are two or more dose combinations with the minimum number of patients, dose combination is randomly selected from them 6. Unless stopping criteria are met, this dose-finding step is continued until the prespecified sample size is reached

(continued)

Table 5.1 (continued)

Method	Phase I/II dose-finding design for two-agent combinations using fixed-reference adaptive randomization	Phase I/II dose-finding design for two-agent combinations using Bayesian moving-reference adaptive randomization	Dose-finding design for two-agent combinations assuming partially ordered dose–toxicity and dose–efficacy relationships	Two-stage design based on zone and dose findings for two-agent combination phase I/II trials
Reference	Huang et al. (2007)	Yuan and Yin (2011a)	Wages and Conaway (2014)	Shimamura et al. (in press)
Stage II dose-finding algorithm	1. Using fixed-reference adaptive randomization (named by Yuan and Yin (2011a)) based on efficacy probability, patients are adaptively randomized to the admissible dose combinations 2. After every cohort of five patients, the prior distributions for the toxicity and efficacy parameters are updated 3. Unless stopping criteria are met, the dose-finding step is continued until the maximum sample size is reached	1. Using Bayesian moving-reference adaptive randomization (named by Yuan and Yin (2011a)) based on efficacy probability, patients are adaptively randomized to the admissible dose combinations 2. After every cohort of five patients, the prior distributions for the toxicity and efficacy parameters are updated 3. Unless stopping criteria are met, dose-finding step is continued until the maximum sample size is reached	1. The dose-finding algorithm at this stage is similar to that of stage I, but the next cohort of patients is allocated the dose combination that has highest efficacy probability estimates among the admissible dose combinations 2. Unless stopping criteria are met, the dose-finding step is continued until the maximum sample size is reached	The admissible dose combinations are chosen based on the estimated toxicity and efficacy probabilities 2. On the basis of the estimated efficacy probabilities for combinations in the admissible dose combinations, a randomization probability is calculated 3. The next cohort of patients is randomized to the combination with this probability among the admissible dose combinations 4. Unless stopping criteria are met, the dose-finding step is continued until the maximum sample size is reached
Early stopping criteria	1. Toxicity (stages I and II) 2. Futility (only stage II) 3. Efficacy (only stage II)	1. Toxicity (stages I and II) 2. Futility (only stage II)	1. Toxicity (stages I and II) 2. Futility (only stage II)	1. Toxicity (stages I and II) 2. Futility (only stage II)

overdose control design. Yuan and Yin (2011b) regarded late-onset toxicities as missing data and proposed an expectation maximization algorithm to account for the unobserved toxicity outcomes in single-agent trials. Liu and Ning (2013) proposed a Bayesian dose-finding design for two-agent combination trials with late-onset toxicities. More recently, some Bayesian phase I/II designs that can address late-onset efficacy and/or toxicity outcomes have been devised (Riviere et al. 2016; Lin and Johnson 2016).

5.3   Accounting for Relative Dose Intensity for MTAs

The conventionally defined RP2D of a cytotoxic agent corresponds to the MTD, which is determined from toxicity data obtained during the first, and rarely, the second cycle of treatment. Toxicity data from later cycles are not used to determine the RP2D; furthermore, treatment changes (e.g., dose reduction or treatment interruption) are recorded but not used to determine the RP2D. Although such a conventional approach has been successful for evaluating cytotoxic agents, it may not be optimal to determine the RP2D of MTAs (Le Tourneau et al. 2010). In this regard, Le Tourneau et al. (2011) recommended that a treatment delay and/or reduction of relative dose intensity be included in the definition of dose limiting toxicity. Relative dose intensity is generally defined as the ratio of the effectively delivered dose to the theoretically administered cumulative dose. Moreover, there are patients who develop chronic low-grade toxicities from MTAs during the evaluation period of phase I trials. Such events eventually warrant a dose reduction or treatment interruption owing to intolerance. The conventional method for determining RP2D relies on the traditional definition of the MTD during cycle 1, wherein low-grade toxicities are not considered and excluded from MTD determination. These toxicities eventually become intolerable and are major factors leading to a dose reduction or interruption after the cycle 1 evaluation period, resulting in insufficient drug exposure. Development of a methodology to predict an appropriate RP2D, instead of basing it on a simple MTD determination, has been advocated. A recent workshop examined Food and Drug Administration (FDA)-approved agents for oncological indications requiring dose reductions and interruptions in initial registration trials for small-molecule kinase inhibitors (Jänne et al. 2016). Among 31 approved inhibitors, at least eight necessitated postmarketing requirements or commitments. There is a significant gap in the development of these agents because of a failure to predict an appropriate administration dose, potentially leading to late-onset and/or cumulative toxicity (Nie et al. 2016). Consequently, there is a need to assess the frequency of cases requiring a dose reduction after cycle 1 and to evaluate the duration and degree of dose lowering (i.e., relative dose intensity). Apart from the MTD, a study on toxicity information in phase I trials revealed that moderate and severe toxicities occur regularly after cycle 1, and attention to RP2D determination may be warranted (Postel-Vinay et al. 2014; Hirakawa et al. 2017). It has been suggested that RP2D assessment should incorporate all available information from any cycle, including lower grade toxicities leading to decreased relative dose intensity.

5.4   Cancer Immunotherapy

The effect of cancer immunotherapies is not directly based on the tumor but rather on the immune system. The mechanism of action of immunotherapy is characterized by a cellular immune response followed by potential changes in the tumor burden or patient survival (Hoos 2012). To adequately evaluate the optimal dose of immunotherapies in phase I trials, a new dose-finding method that accounts for these mechanisms is required. To this end, as in the dose-finding methods for MTAs, this new method would benefit from new trial designs that allow for incorporation of low-grade toxicities, late-onset toxicities, and addition of an efficacy endpoint.

Chiou and Burotto (2015) discussed the pseudo-progression of immunotherapy. Delayed clinical responses have also been observed in studies of immunotherapeutic agents, namely, an increase in the total tumor burden is later followed by tumor regression. These findings of pseudo-progression would have been classified prematurely as progressive disease according to historic WHO or RECIST criteria and have prompted the development of immunotherapy-related response criteria (Wolchok et al. 2009). Therefore, when an efficacy endpoint is evaluated in the dose-finding trials for immunotherapy, we may need to consider pseudo-progression when determining the optimal dose. In this regard, Postel-Vinay et al. (2016) reviewed the phase I designs for immunostimulatory monoclonal antibodies targeting immune checkpoint molecules, including pharmacokinetic and pharmacodynamic evaluations.

5.5   Dose Individualization

An emerging approach among treatments targeted to the needs of individual patients on the basis of genetic, biomarker, phenotypic, or other clinical (or clinicopathological) characteristics is given a great deal of attention (Collins and Varmus 2015). This growing trend is also recognized in early-phase dose-finding trials that determine the RP2D that often corresponds to the MTD defined as the highest clinically safe dose. Several recent dose-finding trials have enrolled two or three heterogeneous groups of patients categorized based on clinical or genomic characteristics (e.g., Innocenti et al. 2014). Such trials were aimed at determining the individualized RP2D for each patient group. To accommodate this growing trend, several dose-finding methods have been developed to identify each RP2D in two or three groups of patients (e.g., O'Quigley et al. 1999; Ivanova and Wang 2006). Nevertheless, a common limitation of these methods is that they can accommodate only a couple of patients' characteristics in the dose–toxicity and/or dose–efficacy models because of the difficulty with estimating model parameters at a limited sample size of early-phase trials; therefore, these methods do not include an interaction term of the dose and patient covariate in their models.

In recent years, phase I/II trials analyzing the mutations in multiple genes (e.g., mutant or wild type) simultaneously are increasing in number (Amatu et al. 2016). For instance, we have 32 ($=2^5$) patterns of gene mutations when a trial tests five genes; therefore, the parameter estimation for dose–toxicity and/or dose–efficacy models including interaction terms of the dose and gene mutation at a limited sample size can be challenging due to the large number of parameters requiring estimation. Ideally, for each gene mutation pattern, the individualized optimal dose that is defined as the most efficacious dose among the doses with acceptable toxicity should be determined if the toxicity (and/or efficacy) outcome and a gene mutation interact. Recently, Guo and Yuan (2016) struggled with this issue and developed a new dose-finding method for identifying an individualized optimal dose for each gene mutation pattern. They proposed the canonical partial least-square method, which is widely used in high-dimensional data analyses, to extract a small number of components from the covariate matrix consisting of the dose, covariates (i.e., genomic markers), and dose-by-covariate interactions. Nonetheless, their method cannot identify the gene(s) influencing toxicity and/or efficacy responses because of its methodological nature: the toxicity and efficacy outcomes are modeled based on a latent variable approach involving the canonical partial least-square components. A dose-finding method that determines the individualized optimal dose for each pattern of multiple patient covariates of interest and then identifies the covariates associated with toxicity and/or efficacy outcomes is needed in practice. This is because the associated covariates are useful for enriching the study population that can be expected to offer a reasonable benefit/risk balance for an investigational drug in subsequent trials.

To accommodate this growing trend, we need to develop a new method for dose individualization and simultaneous covariate selection in early-phase trials evaluating multiple patient covariates of interest. We possibly can create such methods by means of the Bayesian least absolute shrinkage and a selection operator (lasso) (Park and Casella 2008). The Bayesian lasso enables simultaneous parameter estimation and covariate selection in the data with a large number of covariates by shrinking the coefficients of covariates toward zero. For both binary efficacy and toxicity outcomes, the method assumes the logistic model including the dose, binary patient covariates, and interaction of the dose and patient covariates. The logistic model for the efficacy outcome also includes a quadratic term of the dose to enable capturing the nonmonotonic dose–efficacy relationship. The dose assignment during the trial is performed via the posterior distribution of parameters obtained from the Bayesian Lasso. Upon completion of patient enrollment, the proposed method determines the individualized optimal dose according to the patterns of patient covariates and selects the covariates associated with efficacy and toxicity outcomes.

References

Amatu, A., Sartore-Bianchi, A., Siena, S.: NTRK gene fusions as novel targets of cancer therapy across multiple tumour types. ESMO Open **1**, e000023 (2016)

Cheung, Y.K., Chappell, R.: Sequential designs for phase I clinical trials with late-onset toxicities. Biometrics **56**, 1177–1182 (2000)

Chiou, V.L., Burotto, M.: Pseudoprogression and immune-related response in solid tumors. J. Clin. Oncol. **33**, 3541–3543 (2015)

Collins, F., Varmus, H.: A new initiative on precision medicine. New Engl. J. Med. **372**, 793–795 (2015)

Guo, B., Yuan, Y: Bayesian phase I/II biomarker-based dose finding for precision medicine with molecularly targeted agents. J. Am. Stat. Assoc. (2016). https://doi.org/10.1080/01621459.2016.1228534

Hirakawa, A., Yonemori, K., Kinoshita, F., Kobayashi, Y., Ohkuma, H.S., Kawachi, A., Tamura, K., Fujiwara, Y., Rubinstein, L., Harris, P.J., Takebe, N.: Potential utility of a longitudinal relative dose intensity of molecularly targeted agents in phase 1 dose-finding trials. Cancer Sci. (2017). https://doi.org/10.1111/cas.13436

Hoering, A., LeBlanc, M., Crowley, J.: Seamless phase I-II trial design for assessing toxicity and efficacy for targeted agents. Clin. Cancer Res. **17**, 640–646 (2011)

Hoos, A.: Evolution of end points for cancer immunotherapy trials. Ann. Oncol. **23**, 47–52 (2012)

Huang, X., Biswas, S., Oki, Y., Issa, J.-P., Berry, D.A.: A parallel phase I/II clinical trial design for combination therapies. Biometrics **63**, 429–436 (2007)

Innocenti, F., Schilsky, R.L., Ramirez, J., Janisch, L., Undevia, S., House, L.K., Das, S., Wu, K., Turcich, M., Marsh, R., Karrison, T.: Dose finding and pharmacokinetic study to optimize the dosing of irinotecan according to the UGT1A1 genotype of patients with cancer. J. Clin. Oncol. **32**, 2328–2334 (2014)

Ivanova, A., Wang, K.: Bivariate isotonic design for dose-finding with ordered groups. Stat. Med. **25**, 2018–2026 (2006)

Jänne, P.A., Kim, G., Shaw, A.T., Sridhara, R., Pazdur, R., McKee, A.E.: Dose finding of small-molecule oncology drugs: optimization throughout the development life cycle. Clin. Cancer Res. **22**, 2613–2617 (2016)

Le Tourneau, C., Diéras, V., Tresca, P., Cacheux, W., Paoletti, X.: Current challenges for the early clinical development of anticancer drugs in the era of molecularly targeted agents. Target Oncol. **5**, 65–72 (2010)

Le Tourneau, C., Razak, A.R., Gan, H.K., Pop, S., Diéras, V., Tresca, P., Paoletti, X.: Heterogeneity in the definition of dose-limiting toxicity in phase 1 cancer clinical trials of molecularly targeted agents: a review of the literature. Eur. J. Cancer **47**, 1468–1475 (2011)

Lin, S., Johnson, V.E.: A robust Bayesian dose-finding design for phase I/II clinical trials. Biostatistics **17**, 249–263 (2016)

Liu, S., Ning, J.: A Bayesian dose-finding design for drug combination trials with delayed toxicities. Bayesian Anal. **8**, 703–722 (2013)

Mauguen, A., Le Deley, M.C., Zohar, S.: Dose-finding approach for dose escalation with overdose control considering incomplete observations. Stat. Med. **30**, 1584–1594 (2011)

Muler, J.H., McGinn, C.J., Normolle, D., Lawrence, T., Brown, D., Hejna, G., Zalupski, M.M.: Phase I trial using a time-to-event continual reassessment strategy for dose escalation of cisplatin combined with gemcitabine and radiation therapy in pancreatic cancer. J. Clin. Oncol. **22**, 238–243 (2004)

Nie, L., Rubin, E.H., Mehrotra, N., Pinheiro, J., Fernandes, L.L., Roy, A., Bailey, S., de Alwis, D.P.: Rendering the 3 + 3 design to rest: more efficient approaches to oncology dose-finding trials in the era of targeted therapy. Clin. Cancer Res. **22**, 2623–2639 (2016)

O'Quigley, J., Shen, L.Z., Gamst, A.: Two-sample continual reassessment method. J. Biopharm. Stat. **9**, 17–44 (1999)

Park, T., Casella, G.: The Bayesian lasso. J. Am. Stat. Assoc. **103**, 681–686 (2008)

Postel-Vinay, S., Aspeslagh, S., Lanoy, E., Robert, C., Soria, J.C., Marabelle, A.: Challenges of phase 1 clinical trials evaluating immune checkpoint-targeted antibodies. Ann. Oncol. **27**, 214–224 (2016)

Postel-Vinay, S., Collette, L., Paoletti, X., Rizzo, E., Massard, C., Olmos, D., Fowst, C., Levy, B., Mancini, P., Lacombe, D., Ivy, P., Seymour, L., Le Tourneau, C., Siu, L.L., Kaye, S.B., Verweij, J., Soria, J.C.: Towards new methods for the determination of dose limiting toxicities and the assessment of the recommended dose for further studies of molecularly targeted agents-dose-Limiting Toxicity and Toxicity Assessment Recommendation Group for Early Trials of Targeted therapies, an European Organisation for Research and Treatment of Cancer-led study. Eur. J. Cancer **50**, 2040–2049 (2014)

Postel-Vinay, S., Gomez-Roca, C., Molife, L.R., Anghan, B., Levy, A., Judson, I., De Bono, J., Soria, J.C., Kaye, S., Paoletti, X.: Phase 1 trials of molecularly targeted agents: should we pay more attention to late toxicities? J. Clin. Oncol. **29**, 1728–1735 (2011)

Riviere, M.K., Yuan, Y., Jourdan, J.H., Dubois, F., Zohar, S.: Phase I/II dose-finding design for molecularly targeted agent: plateau determination using adaptive randomization. Stat. Methods Med. Res. (2016). https://doi.org/10.1177/0962280216631763

Shimamura, F., Hamada, C., Matsui, S., Hirakawa, A.: Two-stage approach based on zone and dose findings for two-agent combination phase I/II trials. J. Biopharm. Stat. (in press)

Wages, N.A., Conaway, M.R.: Phase I/II adaptive design for drug combination oncology trials. Stat. Med. **33**, 1990–2003 (2014)

Wolchok, J.D., Hoos, A., O'Day, S., Weber, J.S., Hamid, O., Lebbé, C., Maio, M., Binder, M., Bohnsack, O., Nichol, G., Humphrey, R., Hodi, F.S.: Guidelines for the evaluation of immune therapy activity in solid tumors: immune-related response criteria. Clin. Cancer Res. **15**, 7412–7420 (2009)

Yuan, Y., Yin, G.: Bayesian phase I/II adaptive randomized oncology trials with combined drugs. Ann. Appl. Stat. **5**, 924–942 (2011a)

Yuan, Y., Yin, G.: Robust EM continual reassessment method in oncology dose finding. J. Am. Stat. Assoc. **106**, 818–831 (2011b)

Printed in the United States
By Bookmasters